Fitness CYCLING

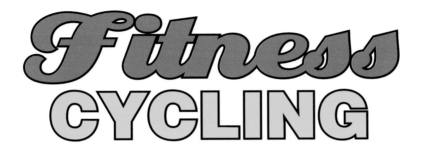

CYCLING

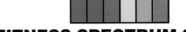

FITNESS SPECTRUM SERIES

Chris Carmichael
Edmund R. Burke

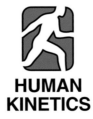

**HUMAN
KINETICS**

Library of Congress Catalog Information

Carmichael, Chris, 1960-
    Fitness cycling / Chris Carmichael, Edmund R. Burke.
        p.   cm. -- (Fitness spectrum series)
    ISBN 0-87322-460-4
    1. Cycling.   2. Physical fitness.   I. Burke, Ed, 1949-   .
    II. Title.   III. Series.
    GV1041.C37 1994   93-42156
    796.6--dc20   CIP

ISBN: 0-87322-460-4

Developmental Editor: Marni Basic; **Assistant Editors:** Sally Bayless, Dawn Roselund, and John Wentworth; **Series Consultant:** Brian Sharkey; **Copyeditor:** Tom Rice; **Proofreader:** Julia Anderson; **Indexer:** Theresa J. Schaefer; **Photo Editor:** Valerie Hall; **Production Director:** Ernie Noa; **Production Manager:** Kris Slamans; **Typesetter:** Ruby Zimmerman; **Text Designer:** Keith Blomberg; **Layout Artists:** Stuart Cartwright and Tara Welsch; **Cover Designer:** Jack Davis; **Photographer (cover, principal interior):** Wilmer Zehr; **Models:** Chuck Mabry, Heidi Selman, cover; Rob Avila, Mike Eastman, Andrea Whitesell, and Al Williamson; **Mac Artists:** Thomas • Bradley and Gretchen Walters; **Illustrator:** Keith Neely; **Printer:** Bang Printing

Human Kinetics books are available at special discounts for bulk purchase. Special editions or book excerpts can also be created to specification. For details, contact the Special Sales Manager at Human Kinetics.

Printed in the United States of America   10   9   8   7   6   5   4   3   2

Human Kinetics
P.O. Box 5076, Champaign, IL 61825-5076
1-800-747-4457

Canada: Human Kinetics, Box 24040, Windsor, ON N8Y 4Y9
1-800-465-7301 (in Canada only)

Europe: Human Kinetics, P.O. Box IW14, Leeds LS16 6TR, England
(44) 532 781708

Australia: Human Kinetics, 2 Ingrid Street, Clapham 5062, South Australia
(08) 371 3755

New Zealand: Human Kinetics, P.O. Box 105-231, Auckland 1
(09) 309 2259

Contents

Part I Preparing to Cycle   1

Chapter 1 Cycling for Fitness   3
Chapter 2 Getting Equipped to Cycle   11
Chapter 3 Checking Your Cycling Fitness   23
Chapter 4 Cycling the Right Way   31
Chapter 5 Warming Up and Cooling Down   39

Part II Cycling Workout Zones   49

Chapter 6 Green Zone   53
Chapter 7 Blue Zone   65
Chapter 8 Purple Zone   79
Chapter 9 Yellow Zone   93
Chapter 10 Orange Zone   105
Chapter 11 Red Zone   119

Part III Training by the Workout Zones   129

Chapter 12 Setting Up Your Program   131
Chapter 13 Sample Cycling Programs   137
Chapter 14 Cross-Training   147
Chapter 15 Charting Your Progress   153

Index   159

About the Authors   165

Credits   167

PART I

PREPARING TO CYCLE

Long thought of as an activity mostly for youth, cycling has become a favorite recreational sport for many of us. Why this popularity? Cycling can be done alone, with a companion, or with a group, for any length of time, at almost any time, and by any reasonably fit person—regardless of age.

Cycling can help you improve your fitness while you enjoy the freedom of the open road or trail. It is one of the best forms of aerobic exercise.

No matter what your cycling experience, you will find something in this book for you. It contains workouts appropriate for all riders—those new to the sport, those who already ride a little but want to add some variety to their cycling, and those who want to discover new cycling options and get more out of their workouts.

Before you undertake any cycling fitness program, it is important to know what the components of fitness are and how to incorporate them into your lifestyle. Chapter 1 describes how your body responds to cycling.

Chapter 2 outlines the basics of choosing equipment to help you get the most out of your training and the type of riding you want to do.

Chapter 3 gives detailed directions for determining your level of fitness and helps you decide what workouts are best for you.

Chapter 4 provides the basics of proper riding technique and body position on the bicycle. Chapter 5 discusses warm-up and cool-down, providing a series of stretching exercises to incorporate into your workouts.

Making a commitment to physical fitness and wellness is one of the most important choices you can make. The first five chapters will help familiarize you with the basics you need to get started in your cycling fitness program. This is the first step on the road to discovering the great feeling of fitness from riding your bicycle.

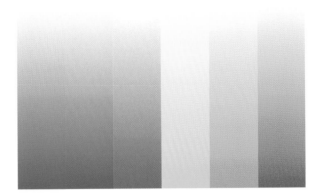

1

Cycling for Fitness

Experts have long recognized bicycling as one of the best forms of aerobic exercise. Almost anyone of any age can cycle for fitness, and anyone in good health can become a proficient rider with practice. Thanks to the efficiency of the bicycle, cycling is an excellent way to build cardiorespiratory and muscular fitness. One of the beauties of bicycling is that you can strengthen your body and your spirits simultaneously. Fun and fitness building go hand in hand.

Even more encouraging is the diversity of the people on bicycles. Those of all ages are working out, racing, or just having a good time. No matter how differently they use their bicycles, riders from the professional cyclist to the weekend tourist have two things in common: they are getting satisfaction from their activity, and they are getting a good workout and burning calories. Everyone who cycles regularly can achieve health and fitness benefits.

That is why this book is so important. As you progress through the 15 chapters, you will learn to solve common problems, refine your technique, and design your own effective and safe cycling fitness program. *Fitness Cycling* is designed to maintain and improve your physical conditioning, one pedal stroke at a time. No matter what your fitness level or cycling ability, we offer a variety of workouts to challenge you. They are designed to help keep your body in motion.

A Sport for Everyone

On any given day, millions of people hop on bicycles and take to city streets, bike paths, and mountain trails. What could be better than whipping down a country road, taking in the beautiful scenery? Cycling can lead you away from a sedentary and stressful lifestyle, and you'll soon discover that it can open up new avenues of fun, fitness, and recreation.

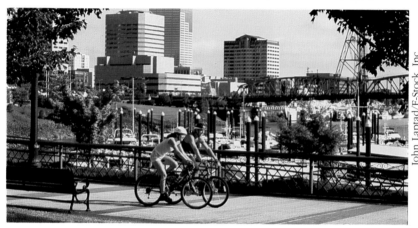

Even in the city, cycling offers a getaway.

More and more cyclists are participating in duathlons (cycling and running), triathlons (cycling, running, and swimming), and competitive road-cycling events. Competitive cycling is a sport that stresses the cardiorespiratory system without putting excess stress on your body's joints.

Millions more people pump the pedals of stationary bicycles at home and at fitness facilities. Although the scenery may not be as good, stationary cyclists get the same physical benefits and don't have to deal with inclement weather or crowded roads. On a stationary bike, you can work out while you watch television, listen to music, or even read the newspaper.

Cycling ranks among the most popular of sporting activities in the United States. The total number of cyclists who exercise regularly is estimated at more than 50 million by the Bicycle Institute of America. The Sporting Goods Manufacturing Association tells us that over 5 million Americans cycle more than 100 days a year. Adults make up 54% of this population, and children under the age of 16 make up 44%. Among adults, 55% of cyclists are women and 45% are men.

One of today's most popular home equipment exercise items is a stationary bicycle—more than 3 million are bought every year. Like many people, you probably do some of your exercising at home. Stationary indoor cycling is an excellent complement to your outdoor cycling.

Fitness is the #1 reason adults give for riding a bicycle. Table 1.1 shows the estimated use of bicycles by various categories based upon 1992 figures.

Table 1.1 Category of Use by Cyclists	
Adults cycling regularly (average once a week)	28 million
Bicycle commuters	4 million
Adults cycling in competition (racing)	240,000
Mountain bike riders	20 million
People touring or vacationing	1.5 million
Recreational event participants (tours, charity rides)	3.5 million

Benefits of Cycling

Bicycling is an excellent way to exercise 20 to 60 minutes a day, 3 to 5 days a week for achieving good health and fitness. Cycling is as effective as walking and running for toning the large muscles of the lower body. It provides the needed aerobic boost to the cardiovascular system but with less stress on your joints.

Aerobic exercise researchers say that cycling is as good as running and swimming for attaining fitness. Sports medicine specialists prescribe cycling because it causes less wear and tear on the joints and muscles than jogging. They often advise older adults and people with joint problems to choose cycling as their primary exercise.

Having selected this book, you probably don't need a lot of convincing that cycling is a worthwhile activity. But a fuller appreciation of how cycling can improve your physical fitness and health can be a constant source of motivation.

Let's look specifically at how cycling can improve each fitness component: cardiovascular fitness, body composition, flexibility, and muscular endurance and strength.

Cardiovascular Fitness

Cycling is one of the best activities for improving cardiovascular fitness. Cardiovascular fitness is measured in terms of aerobic capacity, which is the ability to do large-muscle, whole-body exercise of moderate to high intensity over extended periods of time. Cycling works primarily the muscles of the legs, hips, and buttocks, and the upper body is used during hill climbing. It increases the oxidative capacity of these muscles, thereby improving the body's ability to do extended work.

By engaging in regular vigorous cycling that improves aerobic capacity, you can reduce the risk of heart disease. This kind of activity, called *aerobic exercise*, helps your heart get stronger.

Body Composition

Aerobic cycling several times a week is a fun and fast way to burn fat and calories and increase lean weight. Your body can be divided into two basic components: lean weight (muscle, bone, internal organs) and fat weight. For good health and fitness, you should try to maintain a proper ratio of one to the other. By assessing your body composition, it is possible to determine if you are underweight, muscular, or overweight.

Estimates of body composition are easily determined by measuring skinfolds with calipers. This gives a percentage of body fat, which means that out of a total body weight a certain percentage is estimated to be stored fat. Therefore, if your percentage of fat is 13, the remaining 87% is lean body mass. You should try to maintain body fat below 20% if you are male and below 25% if you are female.

Controlling what you eat (caloric intake) combined with regular aerobic exercise (caloric output) is an ideal way to maintain a balance in body composition. Cycling works all of the major muscle groups of the lower body and can produce a lean, muscular look. Table 1.2 lists the calories burned while cycling at various speeds.

Table 1.2 Calories Burned During Cycling	
Cycling speed (mph)	Calories per mile
10	26
15	31
20	38
25	47
30	59

Flexibility

Flexibility is the ability to move muscles and joints through their full range of motion. Being flexible turns sports like cycling into lifetime activities that can make a real difference in long-term health.

Cycling has very little effect on improving your flexibility. Your goal is to supplement your cycling to avoid what some riders call "cycling rigor mortis"—joint stiffness and gradual loss of muscle elasticity caused by excessive saddle time. Chapter 5 will give you suggestions on how to incorporate stretches into your cycling fitness program for improved performance and for improved overall health.

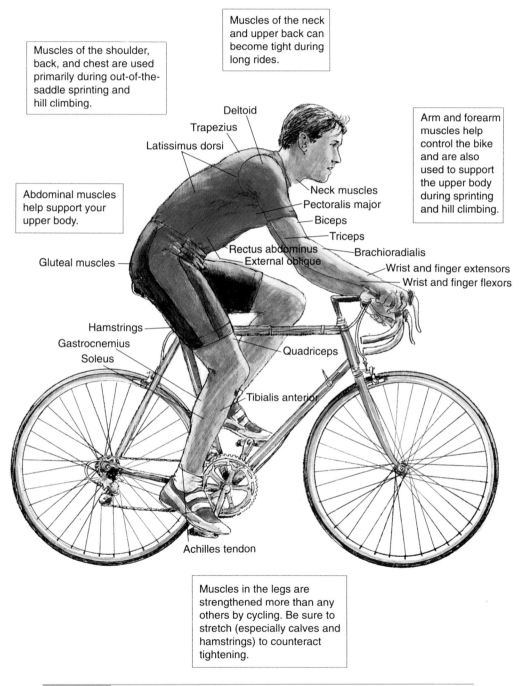

Muscles of the shoulder, back, and chest are used primarily during out-of-the-saddle sprinting and hill climbing.

Muscles of the neck and upper back can become tight during long rides.

Arm and forearm muscles help control the bike and are also used to support the upper body during sprinting and hill climbing.

Abdominal muscles help support your upper body.

Deltoid
Trapezius
Latissimus dorsi
Neck muscles
Pectoralis major
Biceps
Triceps
Rectus abdominus
External oblique
Brachioradialis
Wrist and finger extensors
Wrist and finger flexors
Gluteal muscles
Hamstrings
Gastrocnemius
Soleus
Quadriceps
Tibialis anterior
Achilles tendon

Muscles in the legs are strengthened more than any others by cycling. Be sure to stretch (especially calves and hamstrings) to counteract tightening.

Figure 1.1   Muscles used in cycling.

Muscular Endurance and Strength

Muscular fitness includes both endurance (how many times or how long you can lift or hold an object) and strength (how much weight you can lift). Many activities in your daily life such as lifting grocery bags and walking up several flights of stairs require some degree of muscular fitness.

Cycling enhances muscular strength and endurance, especially for the muscles of the lower body. Figure 1.1 shows how cycling affects the muscles.

For example, a regimen of sprint cycling and riding up hills can strengthen the muscles of the back and shoulders more effectively than some weight-lifting programs. Generally, long-distance, lower-intensity cycling can improve your muscular endurance.

Comparing Cycling's Fitness Benefits

How do the fitness benefits of cycling compare to the benefits of other activities you may want to undertake? How much do you need to cycle to receive the same benefits from cycling as you would from other fitness

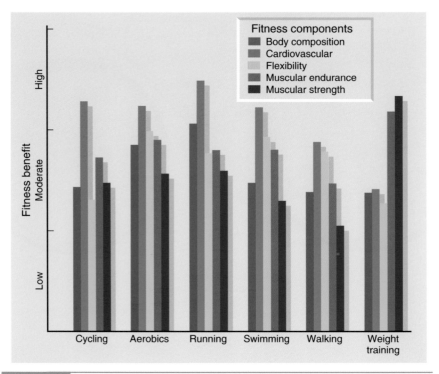

Figure 1.2 How cycling compares to other fitness activities.

activities? Let's compare the aerobic training effect of cycling to that of running and swimming. If you cycle 5 miles in less than 20 minutes, that is comparable to running 1 mile in less than 8 minutes and swimming 600 yards in less than 15 minutes. We can see in Figure 1.2 that cycling compares very well with other sports for the five components of physical fitness.

Cycling is comparable to running, aerobics, and swimming in cardiovascular training, and equal to many activities for maintaining body weight, muscular endurance, and strength.

In addition to the physical benefits of regular aerobic cycling, you can also help increase your sense of well-being and enjoy a more productive and happier life. Kenneth Cooper, author of *Aerobics*, described exercise as "a means of putting more years in your life and more life in your years." As research has shown, even small improvements in fitness—like those achieved through cycling—can substantially reduce the risk of disease.

So don't underestimate the value of getting out and pedaling a bicycle 3 to 5 times a week. Combine a little cycling with other positive lifestyle changes and you have the recipe for better health.

Best of all, cycling is a lifetime activity that can be enjoyed in many different ways. If you are young and full of energy you may want to race, or ride 25 miles in under an hour. If the weather's bad and you want to be fit, you may choose a stationary bike workout. Whatever your needs may be, you'll find a variety of cycling workouts in chapters 6 to 11. In Part III of the book we'll tell you how to incorporate cycling into a fitness program that is right for you. With the help of this book, you should have many great rides—and results—ahead of you.

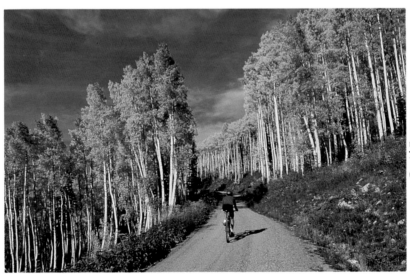

David Epperson

On a bike, you can train almost anywhere.

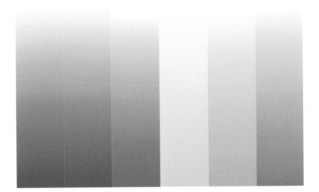

2

Getting Equipped to Cycle

You can still hop on the old 10-speed in your worn pair of tennis shoes, denim shorts, and cotton shirt, but you'll be a lot more comfortable—and therefore more willing to ride—if you invest a little time and money in choosing the right bike and clothing. This chapter will help you make the right selections.

These days you have many choices to make. Do you want a road bike, a mountain bike, or a hybrid? Do you want a basic stationary bike or a sophisticated exercise bike with all the bells and whistles? What cycling wardrobe will you select from the vast array of form-fitting synthetics? What shoes are best for the various forms of cycling?

Choosing a Bike

Having purchased this book, you probably already own a bike. But if you don't, or if you're planning to upgrade, the following sections will help you determine what type of bike is best for you. In searching for a bike, start by deciding what type of riding you want to do. Your local bike shop can provide a focus, but only after you give them the big picture.

Road Bikes

If you plan to stay strictly on the streets, pick a road bike—its light weight, drop bars, and skinny tires are best suited to pounding the pavement over the long haul. Today's road bikes have 14 to 16 speeds, a variety of shifting systems, and weigh about as much as the saddle on your old English racer.

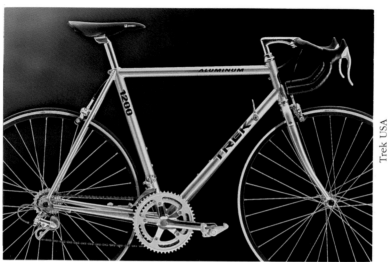

Trek USA

A road bike.

Though mountain bikes account for the lion's share of the bike business these days, a road bike with a 27-inch or a 700c wheel is probably the best all-around fitness machine. The drop-style handlebars give you better aerodynamics and more hand positions—which can help you avoid fatigue and discomfort on long rides—than the straight bars of a mountain bike. The road bike's light weight and narrow tires mean less rolling resistance than a fat-tired mountain bike, but also a less forgiving ride, especially on pavement or dirt roads. Although the gearing range of a road bike is narrower than that of a mountain bike, with a larger "big gear" and a less-accommodating low gear, you don't need the extensive low-gear range a mountain bike offers unless you're planning a loaded-panniers tour of the Rocky Mountains. You will, however, welcome the road bike's bigger gears on long descents.

The biggest drawbacks to buying a road bike are price and choice. Road bikes account for a much smaller share of the market than mountain bikes, so they generally cost more and offer fewer models to choose from.

Mountain Bikes

If you expect to ride mostly off-road, pick a mountain bike. You'll be in good company—6 of every 10 bikes sold in the United States are mountain bikes. With their broad range of gearing and fat, low-pressure tires, mountain bikes are great for pedaling up and down dirt roads and trails. Although they are designed for off-road use, their upright riding style and 26-inch wheels—reminiscent of the old beach cruisers and paperboy bikes from which they are descended—have made them a hit with newcomers to cycling and street riders who find them ideal for pedaling through the urban wilderness.

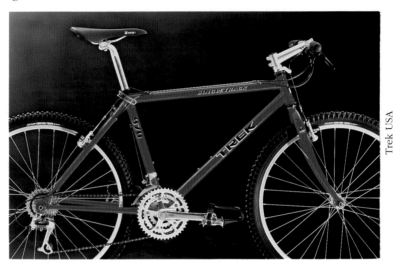

Trek USA

A mountain bike.

If you choose a mountain bike, you'll get fewer flats, thanks to the wide, heavy tires, and you'll stop faster, courtesy of the motorcycle-style cantilever brakes. But you'll also find the upright position, extra weight, and beefy rubber a hindrance on long rides.

There's a wide variety of mountain bikes, ranging from inexpensive steel bikes to top-dollar titanium trail tamers with front and rear suspension.

Hybrids

If you plan to ride both road and trail but don't want to buy two bikes, you might consider buying a hybrid—a bike designed for both road and off-road riding. The hybrid bike is a legitimate choice for riders who want a little dirt (or a little asphalt) in their cycling diets. The tires are wider than road bike tires but narrower than mountain bike tires, and they are often on road-sized (27-inch or 700c) wheels. Although you can use a hybrid on road or trail, its straight bars and upright position aren't really suited for prolonged road rides, and its bigger wheels and narrower tires put technical trails out of reach for most riders. Still, many people who want a taste of both cycling worlds find them an acceptable compromise.

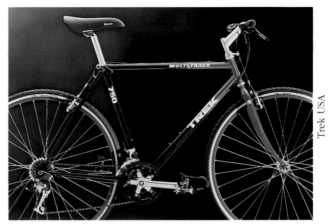

A hybrid bike.

Buying a Bike

Even if you think you've found the bike of your dreams, don't buy it without taking it for a test ride. What you find to be minor annoyances in a 15-minute ride can become major headaches on longer rides. So, save yourself some money and aggravation by test riding a few bikes before buying one. After a number of test rides, one or two bikes will feel right to you.

Borrow bikes from your friends, and ask them for the names of a few reputable dealers. Tell the salesperson what kind of riding you plan to do, ask for some help selecting your proper frame size, then insist that the bikes you test ride be adjusted to provide your optimal riding position—or as close as you can get to it without equipment changes. You'll have to live with your test bikes' stem lengths, for example, but you can fine-tune the saddle's height, angle, and fore-and-aft position. Follow these two rules of thumb:

1. Stand astride your test bike and measure the distance between the top tube and your crotch. You need 1 inch of clearance over the top tube for a road bike or hybrid, and 2 or more inches for a mountain bike.
2. While in the riding position, the handlebars and stem should block your view of the front wheel's hub.

If you are undecided about two frame sizes, it's usually best to choose the smaller size. It is critical for both safety and comfort to have the right size frame when cycling.

What to Spend

Bike prices range from just under $250 for a steel bike with no-frills components to $4,000 and up for elite steeds combining the latest frame materials and the best components. If you want a good, lively bike with quality components, expect to pay about $400 to $600 for a hybrid, $500 to $750 for a mountain bike, or $600 to $900 for a road bike.

It's a buyer's market when it comes to exercise or stationary bikes. The products offered to consumers are diverse. A quality indoor bicycle can be purchased for slightly more than $300. Quality bikes will give you an accurate reading of resistance so that you can repeat a workout and calculate the calories burned. With less expensive bikes you have to estimate the tension. Most of the quality exercise bikes range in price between $300 and $700, and computerized models can range from $1,000 to $4,000.

One way to have the best of both worlds is to buy a wind trainer ($100 to $300 or more). These indoor trainers use your bicycle and fans, magnets, or a combination of the two to provide resistance. You attach your bike to the trainer, then use your bike's gears to determine the degree of resistance. As with other indoor trainers, some versions are basic and others are computerized.

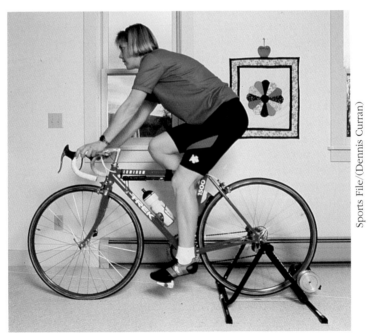

Sports File/(Dennis Curran)

Indoor trainers offer the same physical benefits as riding on the road.

Accessories and Gear

Once you've found a bike to ride you may think you're done shopping, but we suggest you purchase a few items to make your cycling a lot safer and more comfortable.

Helmets

Your second major purchase should be a helmet meeting Snell, ANSI, or ASTM standards. Unlike their heavy, hard-shelled predecessors, today's lightweight expanded-polystyrene helmets weigh less than a half pound, provide ventilation to keep your head cool, and cost as little as $30—a small cost for the valuable protection they provide.

Some helmets blend internal plastic mesh with a Lycra cover; others employ a lightweight, hard-shell coating. All are designed to distribute and thus minimize the force of an impact. Make sure the salesperson shows you how to get a proper fit—a loose helmet is almost as bad as none at all. Most come in three standard sizes—small, medium, and large—and rely on removable pads to provide the custom fit each head requires. Never wear a helmet once it's been damaged in a spill. Many manufacturers will provide a replacement at little or no cost.

Padded Shorts

Next on your list of cycling accessories is a pair of good-quality cycling shorts. You'll find the smooth padding provided by the synthetic chamois liner much more comfortable than the seam running down the center of your old pair of cutoffs. These nylon-and-Lycra garments have a high back, designed to fit a body that's leaned over on a bike, and their length keeps your thighs from rubbing on the saddle. Elastic on the lower leg helps keep them from riding up while you're riding along. Some shorts designed for off-road riding even have hip and thigh pads to offer protection in the event of a spill.

Prices vary depending on quality, but you can expect to pay between $25 and $75. Consider buying at least two pairs, so you can wear one while the other is in the wash—riding in dirty shorts can lead to unpleasant bacterial invasions called *saddle sores* that are every bit as unpleasant as they sound. One way to minimize the likelihood of these eruptions is to rub the liner with vitamin A & D ointment, which also helps keep both real and synthetic chamois soft and pliable. Another is to wash occasionally with an antibacterial soap, such as Betadine. A third strategy is to remove your shorts as soon as possible after a ride.

Gloves

Your third purchase should be a pair of fingerless cycling gloves. These pad your hands where they contact the handlebars, a welcome buffer against some of the bumpy roads you're sure to encounter, and because your fingers aren't covered you retain the delicate control needed on shifting and brake levers. They also absorb sweat, giving you a better grip on the bars, and will protect your palms in the event of a spill, when your natural reaction will be to throw your hands out to catch yourself. It's much easier—and a good deal less painful—to buy a new pair of gloves than to wait for your palms to recover from a severe case of road rash. Expect to pay $15 to $30 for good gloves, and keep an eye out for a design that has a terrycloth thumb—it's handy for wiping the sweat away on a hot day.

Shoes

Finally, buy yourself a pair of cycling shoes. You may think running shoes are an acceptable compromise, but this is one purchase where half-stepping just won't do. The sole of a running shoe is too springy for cycling because it's intended to protect the foot as it pounds the ground. Cycling shoes, which make limited contact with the ground, have stiffer soles that help transmit power to the pedals—indeed, some models can be quite uncomfortable to walk in, even for a short distance.

In general, shoes fall into three categories—touring, racing, and off-road riding. Touring shoes resemble running shoes but have stiffer soles and rudimentary integrated cleats for gripping the pedal; you'll be able to do some walking in these, but don't plan any long hikes. Expect to pay $40 to $60.

Racing, or "cleated," shoes are more efficient for riding but almost useless for walking. Their soles are inflexible and equipped with removable, adjustable cleats designed to work either with standard pedals with toe clips and straps or with clipless pedals that incorporate a binding system similar to that used with skis. With the greater specialization comes a higher price—$60 to $140 and up. If you decide on this type of shoe, make sure your shop helps fit you and your new shoes to your pedals. Although some clipless systems provide a degree of "float" for the foot during the pedal stroke, poorly set-up cleats can lead to knee injuries.

Off-road shoes, which tend to look more like low-top hiking boots, have more rugged soles and some flexibility in the toebox, since they come in contact with the earth more often than their on-road counterparts. Versions are available both for standard and clipless pedals; some shoes can be used with either system. Because many off-road shoes are used for racing as well as riding, they run a little more expensive than touring shoes—$50 to $100 and up. And the caveat about cleat setup applies here, too.

Touring shoes are best for indoor cycling if they are used with toe clips and straps. Toe clips will help keep the ball of your foot centered over the pedals and should be an addition to your stationary bicycle.

Shoes will be one of the most important purchases you make, so take your time picking them out. If you find the choices too confusing, tell your salesperson what kind of riding you plan to do and let her or him fit you with the proper shoe for the job.

Other Essentials

You're going to get thirsty, so add two water bottle cages and water bottles (about $15 for all four items). And you're going to have flats, so pick out a frame pump ($20 and up) and a saddle bag ($10 and up). Fill the last item with tire irons ($2 and up), a patch kit ($2), and at least one spare tube ($5 and up). If you've never fixed a flat, ask the salesperson or a friend to show you how. A handlebar computer ($30 and up) can chart your road to fitness by logging elapsed time, distance, speed, and other information.

For indoor cycling, various accessories are also essential. Don't even consider indoor cycling without a fan. If you don't believe us, just try cycling for 30 minutes on your indoor bike in the summer or spring. You'll work up such a sweat that you will probably not finish the workout. For effective cooling, you need to use something as large as a window fan ($30). Many cyclists consider a reading stand an invaluable accessory, especially if they do not enjoy watching television or listening to music. Several companies make these stands, which attach to the handlebars and begin at about $25.

Optional Accessories

We have described what you must have—now let's look at what you ought to have. The following items aren't indispensable, but they will make your riding more enjoyable.

Jersey.   Cycling jerseys are form-fitting garments blending natural and synthetic fibers that wick perspiration away from your body for rapid evaporation. This helps keep you cool in summer and forestalls hypothermia in winter. Long- and short-sleeve versions are available; all have a front zipper to aid ventilation and two or three rear pockets for carrying keys, extra clothing, and food. Prices range from $30 to $60. Buy two so you'll always have clean clothes for riding. And save your T-shirts for wearing underneath the jersey—if you crash, the two garments will slide against one another, sparing you some scrapes.

Jacket.   It's not always nice outside, and there's nothing worse than pedaling home in a bone-chilling downpour. A lightweight rain jacket is a must for fall and spring rides; most compress easily into a jersey pocket, and some even turn into their own zippered bags. Prices run $40 and up. If you want to keep cycling through the winter, you'll need a heavier garment with a windproof, water-resistant shell. Expect to pay $70 or more.

Tights.   Popularized by aerobic dance classes, tights serve to keep the knees and quads warm when the temperature dips below 60 degrees. You'll generate your own windchill on a frosty day, and a good set of tights will keep those large muscle groups toasty and help prevent knee injuries, the bane of any cycling program. Expect to pay $40 to $70, depending on weight. You may want to buy lightweight tights for chilly days and more insulated tights for wintry weather.

Arm and leg warmers.   These tubelike affairs, like giant socks with no toes, are great for days that are too warm for tights and long-sleeved jerseys, but too cool for shorts and short sleeves. Pull them on at the outset of your ride, and as you warm up, peel down, stuffing the warmers in your pockets. Materials range from Lycra and nylon for cool days to wool for cold or damp days. About $15 to $20.

Eyewear.   Sunglasses will keep bugs and grit out of your eyes while protecting them against ultraviolet and reflected glare. The one-piece design of most cycling sunglasses eliminates airflow through the nose bridge, and their brow pads help keep sweat out of the eyes. Most come with interchangeable lenses designed for a variety of conditions, from bright sun to overcast; some models even accommodate prescription lenses. Expect to pay $70 and up, and more for prescription glasses.

Heart rate monitor.   As you progress in your training, you should seriously consider buying a heart rate monitor to measure your heart rate as you ride. These monitors pick up the electrical activity of your heart and relay it to a receiver mounted on your handlebar. A basic unit that simply tells you your heart rate will cost about $100; others that allow you to set your upper and lower target heart rate zones can be purchased for about $125 to $150.

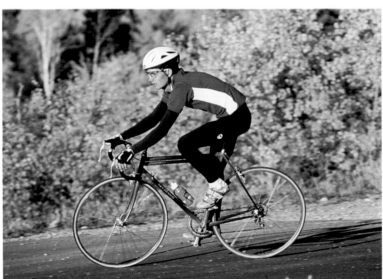

David Epperson

Arm and leg warmers are ideal for cool days.

Adding Up the Costs

How much you will spend on your cycling wardrobe and accessories will depend on whether you purchase only the bare essentials or go all-out.

LOW BUDGET COSTS	
HELMET	$ 35-120
PADDED SHORTS	25-75
GLOVES	15-30
CYCLING SHOES	40-60
WATER BOTTLE AND CAGE	10
FRAME PUMP	20
SADDLE BAG	10
TIRE IRONS, PATCH KIT, SPARE TUBE	10
TOTAL COST	$165-335

Depending on your needs and tastes, you can also spend a little more for basic items or purchase some additional accessories:

HIGH BUDGET COSTS	
HELMET	$ 35-120
PADDED SHORTS (2 PAIR)	50-150
GLOVES	15-30
CLEATED SHOES	60-140
WATER BOTTLES AND CAGES	20
FRAME PUMP	20
SADDLE BAG	10
TIRE IRONS, PATCH KIT, SPARE TUBE	10
JERSEY	30-60
JACKET	40-80
TIGHTS	40-70
ARM & LEG WARMERS	15-20
EYEWEAR	70 AND UP
HEART RATE MONITOR	100-150
TOTAL COST	$ 515-950

Don't be surprised by the cost of these items. With the exception of spare inner tubes, riding gear is built to last and won't need replacing often.

Picking a Road

Look for wide roads with paved shoulders, few stop signs or traffic lights, and a minimum of traffic. Your local cycling club can give you some pointers here—and chances are they conduct some regular training rides that you can join.

Four-lane roads give motorists the option of changing lanes. Interstate highways, where bikes are permitted, are not exciting but they have big shoulders.

Picking a Trail or Dirt Road

Almost any dirt road will do for a fat-tire excursion, but look for those with low traffic—nothing takes your mind off your workout like a faceful of dust and rocks thrown up by passing autos. Many trails are open to bikes, but some are not; they're usually marked as such and should be avoided. Be especially wary of trails frequented by equestrians because horses are not fond of bicycles (some speculate that the buzzing of derailleurs reminds horses of a rattlesnake's warning rattle). Again, your local cycling club can help here and may conduct regular off-road training rides.

Obey the Law

Most cities, counties, and states require cyclists to follow the same rules made for other vehicle operators; some add a few special requirements. In general,

- ride with traffic, not against it, and as far to the right as is practical;
- signal your turns, and be predictable in your movements; don't wander right and left, but keep to a straight line;
- obey all traffic laws as if you were driving your car—that means stopping for red lights and stop signs, yielding to merging traffic, and turning from the proper lanes.

If you're riding off road, follow these guidelines:

- Strive not to damage trails by skidding through corners and descents or spinning out on loose climbs. This accelerates erosion and has led to more than one trail being closed to bikes.
- Announce your presence when you overtake someone (a bell is a nice touch).

- Yield the trail to horses, pedestrians, and other trail users. Don't hammer around blind corners—there may be a hiker coming around the other side.
- Consider taking a day off from time to time to help your local cycling club repair and maintain the area's trail network.

Ride Smart

Think ahead—keep these tips in mind as you head out on your bike:

- Always take at least one water bottle, no matter how short the ride. And drink before you get thirsty—dehydration is a common problem among many cyclists because they don't notice how much they sweat because the breeze they generate evaporates it. Sip frequently, and refill when necessary.
- Take snacks on any ride of 45 minutes or more. Fruit bars, bananas, energy bars, grapes, raisins, orange slices—anything easily digestible will do. Experiment with a variety of snacks.
- Carry extra clothing in your jersey pockets, especially if you live in an area with unpredictable weather. A light rain jacket is a good idea; so are arm and leg warmers, especially in early spring or late fall. Slip some change in there, too, in case you have a mishap and need to phone home, and keep $5 in your seat pack in case you need to buy food, energy drink, or a spare tube to fix a flat.
- When possible, begin your ride into the wind—this may give you a tailwind on the way home, which can be especially welcome after a long, hard ride.

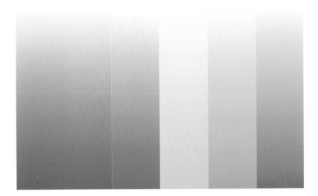

3

Checking Your Cycling Fitness

Before you begin using the workout programs introduced in this book, we want you to answer a few questions about your current fitness and health. Many health benefits are associated with regular cycling. Completing this checklist is a sensible first step toward increasing your physical activity. It will tell you whether you are ready for a cycling self-test and with what level of training you may want to experiment. For many of us, physical activity poses no problem or hazard. This cycling readiness questionnaire is designed to identify the small number of people who should seek medical advice about the extent and activity most suitable for them.

Test Your Health/Fitness

Before you begin the specific programs outlined in chapters 6 to 11, take a few minutes to answer the following questions. Here we offer a self-test that is specific to cycling. It checks both your health history and your fitness habits.

Choose the number that best describes you in each of these 10 areas, then add up your score. The results tell whether your starting line condition is high, average, or low.

ASSESSING YOUR CYCLING FITNESS

Cardiovascular Health

Which of these statements best describes your cardiovascular condition? This is a critical safety check before you enter any vigorous activity. (*Warning:* If you have such a disease history, start the cycling programs in this book only after receiving clearance from your doctor—and then only with close supervision by a fitness instructor.)

No history of heart disease or circulatory
problems   _____ (3)

Past ailments have been treated successfully   _____ (2)

Such problems exist but no treatment required   _____ (1)

Under medical care for cardiovascular disease   _____ (0)

Injuries

Which of these statements best describes your current injuries? This is a test of your musculoskeletal readiness to start a cycling program. (*Warning:* If your injury is temporary, wait until it is cured before starting the program. If it is chronic, adjust the program to fit your limitations.)

No current injury problems   _____ (3)

Some pain in activity but not limited by the
injury   _____ (2)

Level of activity is limited by the injury   _____ (1)

Unable to do much strenuous training   _____ (0)

Illnesses

Which of these statements best describes your current illnesses? Certain temporary or chronic conditions will delay or disrupt your cycling program. (See warning under "Injuries.")

No current illness problems   _____ (3)

Some problem in activity but not limited by it   _____ (2)

Level of activity is limited by the illness   _____ (1)

Unable to do much strenuous training   _____ (0)

(continued)

ASSESSING YOUR CYCLING FITNESS (*continued*)

Age

Which of these age groups describes you? In general, the younger you are, the less time you have spent slipping out of shape.

Age 20 or younger	_____ (3)
Ages 21 to 29	_____ (2)
Ages 30 to 39	_____ (1)
Ages 40 and older	_____ (0)

Weight

Which of these figures describes how close you are to your own definition of ideal weight? Excess fat is a major indicator of unfitness, but it's also possible to be significantly underweight.

At or very near ideal body weight	_____ (3)
Less than 10 pounds above or below the ideal	_____ (2)
10 to 19 pounds above or below ideal weight	_____ (1)
20 or more pounds above or below the ideal	_____ (0)

Resting Pulse Rate

Which of these figures describes your current pulse rate on waking up in the morning but before getting out of bed? A well-trained heart beats slower and more efficiently than one that's unfit.

Below 60 beats per minute	_____ (3)
60 to 69 beats per minute	_____ (2)
70 to 79 beats per minute	_____ (1)
80 or more beats per minute	_____ (0)

Smoking

Which of these statements best describes your smoking history and current habit (if any)? Smoking is the #1 enemy of health and fitness.

Never a smoker	_____ (3)
Once a smoker but quit	_____ (2)
An occasional, light smoker now	_____ (1)
A regular, heavy smoker	_____ (0)

(*continued*)

ASSESSING YOUR CYCLING FITNESS (*continued*)

Most Recent Cycling Outing

Which of these statements best describes your cycling within the last month? The best measure of how well you will cycle in the near future is what you cycled in the past.

Cycled nonstop for more than 1 hour _____ (3)

Cycled nonstop for 30 minutes to 1 hour _____ (2)

Cycled nonstop for less than 30 minutes _____ (1)

No recent bicycle ride of any distance _____ (0)

Cycling Background

Which of these statements best describes your cycling history? Cycling fitness isn't long-lasting, but the fact that you once cycled is a good sign that you can do it again.

Trained for cycling within the past year _____ (3)

Trained for cycling within 1 to 2 years ago _____ (2)

Trained for cycling more than 2 years ago _____ (1)

Never trained formally for cycling _____ (0)

Related Activities

Which of these statements best describes your participation in other exercises that are similar to cycling in their aerobic benefit? The closer they relate to cycling (cross-country skiing, in-line skating, running, for example), the better the carryover effect will be.

Regularly practice similar aerobic activities _____ (3)

Regularly practice less vigorous aerobics _____ (2)

Regularly practice nonaerobic sports _____ (1)

Not regularly active in any physical activity _____ (0)

TOTAL SCORE _____

If you scored 20 points or more, you rate high in health and fitness for a beginning cyclist. You can probably handle continuous rides lasting 45 minutes or longer at an easy to moderate pace.

Between 10 and 19 points, your score is average. You may need to take a break or two to complete a 45-minute ride.

A score of less than 10 points is below average. You may need to start cycling slowly, or start your program on a stationary bicycle where you can take breaks off the bicycle.

Test Your Cycling Fitness

Knowledge of your physical fitness level before you begin using the workout zones in Part II can help you start at an appropriate level and set reasonable goals. Your overall health assessment level also provides a baseline against which you can compare subsequent tests as you progress.

Now comes your final exam. This is the most telling of tests, because up to now you've only surveyed your health and fitness with pen and paper. Now you check it where it counts—on the bike. Based on your performance in this test, you will be able to design an exercise program that is right for you.

The cycling efficiency test can provide you with an accurate determination of your fitness level. It offers you a safe way to determine which workout zones to use for effective and challenging cardiovascular exercise. The test can be used by any age group and at any level of fitness, and it only requires your bicycle and a level riding course.

CYCLING EFFICIENCY TEST

1. Locate a measured 3-mile course at a convenient location (perhaps a residential area of town, a large city park, or a mall parking lot). It can be a straight-out course or a series of loops that make up the 3 miles.
2. Stretch and warm up for 5 to 10 minutes (see chapter 5). You should also be dressed comfortably and have your bicycle properly adjusted.
3. Choose a day when the wind is relatively calm and the temperature is not very high. It may be best to perform this test in the early morning or evening, when environmental conditions are usually more favorable.
4. Do not eat for at least 2 hours before your test, and don't participate in vigorous activity the day before.
5. Ride the 3-mile course as fast as you can, maintaining a steady pace. Time your ride to the nearest second. Pace yourself so you can ride the course at a steady pace for the whole distance; if you need to stop or slow way down, keep your watch running during all breaks. Record your time.
6. The time it takes you to complete the 3-mile course will give you an estimate of your relative fitness level. This will help you design your training program.

Fitness category	Minutes for 3-mile ride
Males	
Below average	More than 12 minutes
Moderately fit	8 to 12 minutes
Highly fit	Less than 8 minutes
Females	
Below average	More than 15 minutes
Moderately fit	11 to 15 minutes
Highly fit	Less than 11 minutes

For example, if you are a male cyclist and you ride the 3 miles in 11 minutes and 45 seconds, you are in the moderately-fit category. Remember, this is your *current* cycling fitness level and says nothing about your potential.

1-4-16 11.51 in 3 miles 15 Ave SFC

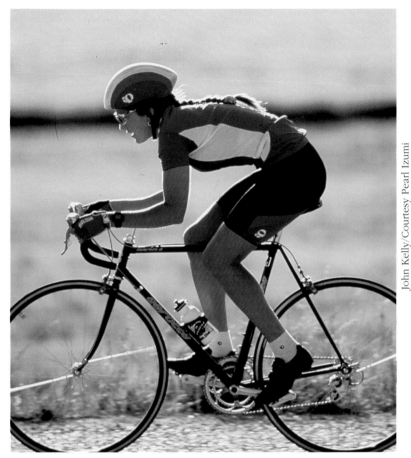

Ride the test as fast as you can, but maintain a steady pace.

John Kelly/Courtesy Pearl Izumi

Retesting

You can retest yourself periodically using this 3-mile cycling efficiency test to establish your gains in performance and fitness. You can retest as often as once a month or on a quarterly basis. To compare cycling efficiency tests, you should ride on the same course, with similar environmental conditions and with comparable bicycles.

No matter what you scored on the cycling efficiency test, you'll find a variety of workouts in Part II that correspond to your current fitness level. You will also find sample programs in chapter 13 that are right for you, no matter what your fitness level or goals.

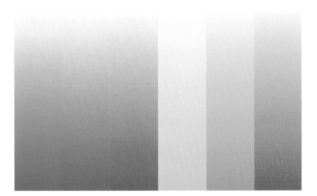

4

Cycling the Right Way

The secret to cycling efficiently is a smooth, relaxed pedaling style that creates a flow that will eat up the miles. But this won't happen if your bicycle does not fit or if you don't pedal correctly. This chapter will introduce you to proper position on a bike and how to pedal your bicycle correctly.

There's more to making your bike fit than adjusting the seat height. Proper positioning on a bicycle can provide benefits you probably haven't thought about. You'll feel much more relaxed and refreshed at the end of a day's ride.

Little aches and pains you may now take for granted could be eliminated with careful bicycle setup and pedaling technique. Since you won't be fighting discomfort, you'll ride farther and faster. And you won't be as vulnerable to possible overuse injuries.

Adjusting Your Bike

When you experiment with the following changes, make one adjustment at a time so you can feel what effect it has. And remember, it takes time to get used to a new position. Ride for several days with this new position before you decide whether a change is right or not.

Saddle Height

The saddle height is the most important adjustment you can make on your bicycle. Proper adjustment allows for efficient use of your muscles and ensures greater comfort while cycling. The directions for saddle height fit all three varieties of bicycles. After you have adjusted the saddle height, make sure that at least 2-1/2 inches of seat post remain in the seat tube for safety. Most seat posts have a maximum height mark on the post; do not exceed this amount.

The height of your saddle is based on your inseam length. Your saddle is correctly positioned when you are sitting squarely on the saddle with your down leg fully extended and the heel of your cycling shoe touching the pedal comfortably. The crankarm should be in line with the seat tube, and someone should be holding the seat from behind to help balance you and the bike. Using your heel to set the height will ensure a slight bend in your knee when you pedal with the ball of your foot. Do not pedal with your heel. Your saddle should be level or slightly tilted with the front of the saddle higher than the rear.

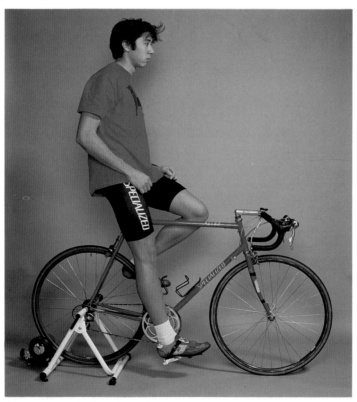

Adjusting saddle height.

Once the saddle height is correct, front and back positioning can be adjusted on the bicycle. While someone is holding your saddle from the back, put both feet into the pedals with the ball of the foot over the pedal axle, and move the pedals to a level position. Drop a plum line from the center of the knee (behind the knee cap); the string should fall directly in line with the pedal axle. The saddle should be moved forward or backward until the plumb line hits the axle. With your knee lined up over the pedal, you can use the muscles of your upper leg to pedal efficiently.

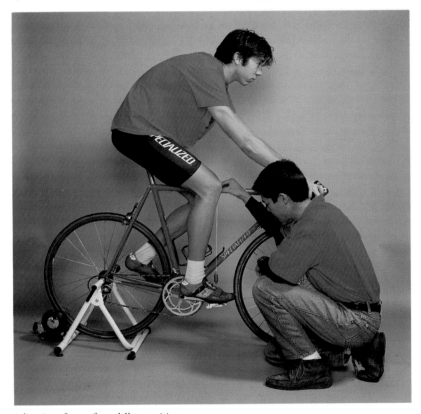

Adjusting fore-aft saddle position.

Please keep in mind that if you make large adjustments to the fore or aft position, you may have to check seat height again. Moving the saddle forward is the same as moving the saddle down; moving the saddle back in effect raises the saddle.

Handlebar Adjustment

On your road or touring bicycle with dropped handlebars, the top of the stem should be level to 1-1/2 inches below the top of your saddle. On your mountain or hybrid bicycle, the top of the handlebars should be at the top of your saddle or slightly lower.

Like your seat post, there is a maximum height that your stem should be extended out of the steering head tube (head set). Usually there is a maximum height mark stamped on the handlebar stem.

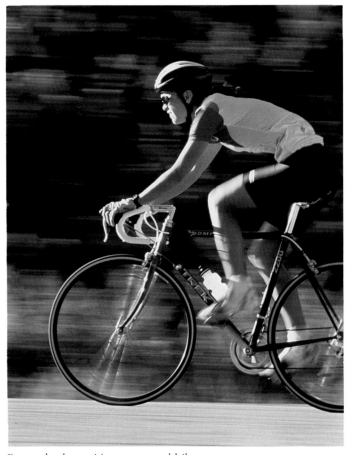

Kevin Syms/F-Stock, Inc.

Proper body position on a road bike.

Stem length is the hardest dimension to prescribe because everyone has different back flexibility and upper-body musculature. In general, your stem should be long enough so that the crossbar of the handlebar obscures the front hub when you are seated and your hands are on the break hoods of a road bicycle or on the grips of a mountain or hybrid bicycle. As you gain experience, consider changing to a longer stem to flatten your back and to improve your aerodynamics. Always ride with your elbows flexed slightly; you can better absorb the bumps and vibration of the road, and you will have less fatigue in your arms, neck, and shoulders.

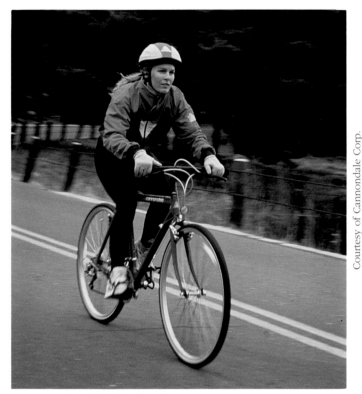

Courtesy of Cannondale Corp.

Proper body position on a mountain bike or hybrid.

Pulling It All Together

These pointers, of course, are not the last word on fitting yourself on a bicycle. Fitting for the professional cyclist is a complex process that can take up to several months to complete.

If you already own a bicycle, have someone at your local bicycle shop help you, or contact your local bike club for assistance.

Although these adjustments may not seem to affect you immediately, give them time. The more time and miles you put on your bicycle, the more you will appreciate a well-fitted bicycle.

The same adjustments should be made on your stationary bicycle if you plan to buy one for home use. If you use one at a health club, make sure your seat height is set properly.

Riding Correctly

After you have adjusted your bicycle, you need to learn about gearing and pedaling cadence (how fast you pedal, expressed in revolutions per minute, or RPM) to ensure comfort and efficiency, and to put less stress on knee joints.

Pedaling and Gearing

Inexperienced cyclists have a tendency to pedal in gears that are much too high for them, and in a cadence that is far too low. Beginning cyclists should strive to pedal at about 70 RPM. Pedaling cadence can easily be timed by counting the down stroke of one foot for a 15-second period and then multiplying the total by 4.

By maintaining a high revolution rate with a relatively low gear ratio, less muscle strength is required and endurance is increased. In contrast, pedaling in a high gear at a low cadence requires significantly more strength and puts undue stress on the knees and hip joints, which can lead to injuries.

After several weeks, begin to raise your cadence until you can pedal consistently in the 85 to 100 RPM range. Experienced cyclists prefer to ride at these higher cadences. It may take up to 6 months or more before you can pedal comfortably at this cadence.

At first, you may find that raising your cadence seems too fast and literally throws you around on the seat. However, with practice a cadence of 85 or greater can be enjoyable and relaxing.

The Importance of Shifting

To help you maintain a high RPM, you should shift gears when necessary. As the terrain or wind varies, you should switch to a higher or lower gear whenever you feel your cadence is too fast or too slow. Figure 4.1 shows gearing on a road bike.

Work with your local bicycle shop to ensure that you have the proper gears on your bicycle to ride comfortably and efficiently in the area where you live. You can purchase replacement chainrings or rear gears.

The terrain you travel should determine the range of gears you'll use. If you live in a hilly area, you'll use lower gears; in a flat area you'll use higher gears. If you live in an area with varied topography, you'll need to be proficient in switching gears.

Learn to shift to a higher gear when you "spin out" (can't keep up with the pedals) and to a lower gear when your RPMs drop. If you consciously do this, it will become automatic; it will also smooth out your pedal stroke and ultimately save you from the pain created by the stress put on your knees by the low RPM pedaling and high torque.

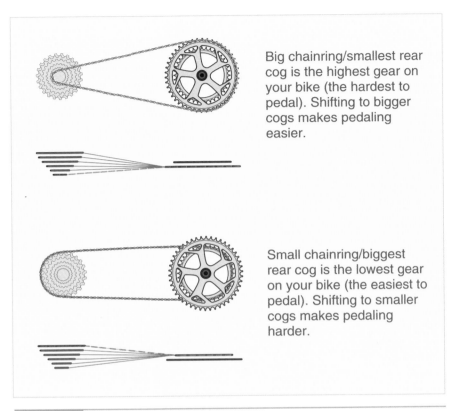

Big chainring/smallest rear cog is the highest gear on your bike (the hardest to pedal). Shifting to bigger cogs makes pedaling easier.

Small chainring/biggest rear cog is the lowest gear on your bike (the easiest to pedal). Shifting to smaller cogs makes pedaling harder.

Figure 4.1   Gearing on a road bike.

What Counts

For proper handling, comfort, and efficient pedaling technique, you need to be properly fitted to your bicycle. Your position on the bike is the most important factor for a smooth ride.

The art of riding your bicycle is largely how you pedal. Having your position set correctly, pedaling smoothly, and riding in the right gear lets you ride easier. The result is comfort and improved performance, and this is the basis for riding for long periods of time.

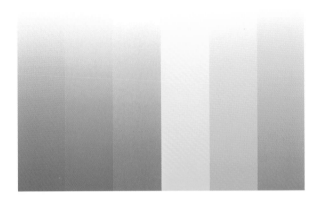

5

Warming Up and Cooling Down

One of the most appealing aspects of cycling is that it is easy on the body—no pounding, no range of motion extremes, no adverse twisting. Just sit on the bicycle and spin the pedals.

With all the physiological accolades given to cycling, you may wonder why you should bother warming up, stretching, and cooling down. Some cyclists figure they can hop on a bicycle and begin an intense workout without any preparation. Besides, who wants to spend time riding easy and stretching when you could be out riding?

Warming Up

Warming up is a term used to describe a variety of activities—calisthenics, stretching, or easy cycling, for example—performed to prepare your body for prolonged physical activity, such as cycling.

We strongly recommend using a warm-up to enhance your cycling performance. A warm muscle contracts more quickly; oxygen is better delivered to the muscles of the legs, back, and upper body; and metabolic rate is increased.

Considerable research has been conducted on the best way to warm up. Active warm-up involves muscle activity, and passive warm-up involves warming the muscles through external means such as massage or sauna. Passive warm-up, however, is less likely to warm the deep muscles. Also, passive warm-up can be counterproductive. By increasing the surface temperature of the skin and dilating blood vessels, passive warm-up diverts a large amount of blood to the skin rather than to the cycling muscles of your legs.

A good warm-up helps prevent injury and makes your cycling workouts easier. Your body does not like to go suddenly from a state of rest to high-intensity activity. The smoother the adjustment, the easier your body adapts to the cycling workout, especially when exercising in the more difficult zones.

What's the Best Way to Warm Up?

The most effective warm-up consists of riding your bicycle. Begin by riding at a slow, gentle pace, then build gradually to your target heart intensity (the pace at which you'll do the main part of your workout). You may also want to do some brisk walking before you get on the bicycle. You can also begin by riding a stationary bike, or by jogging or walking. Try to involve both the arms and the legs in the warm-up.

How Long Should a Warm-Up Last?

You're probably warmed up if you're just beginning to sweat. If you don't reach a sweat, you should at least feel warm, and the exercise should start to feel easier. This usually occurs in about 5 to 10 minutes. Your heart rate should reach about 90 to 110 beats per minute, depending on your age. You should not feel fatigued after warming up.

The Role of Stretching

Stretching should begin after you have warmed up on the bicycle for a few minutes. If warming up on the bike is inconvenient, do some brisk walking or calisthenics for a few minutes. Stretching while the muscles are not warmed up does little to increase the elasticity of your muscles and joints. Raising the temperature of the muscles is a more effective way to increase muscle elasticity.

The Cool Part of the Workout

The cool-down is not as widely practiced as the warm-up, but it is no less important. Casual athletes, in particular, tend to ignore the importance of cooling down. Your cool-down is a period of low-intensity cycling that follows a moderate or vigorous workout, and it lasts about 5 minutes. A cool-down is like a warm-up in reverse. While a warm-up helps your cardiovascular system and muscles to get into gear, a cool-down helps them return gradually to a resting level.

Why Cool Down?

If you stop cycling abruptly, the blood "pools" in the wide-open blood vessels of the legs. Not enough blood returns to the heart, so the heart attempts to beat faster to increase the flow. You may begin to feel light-headed as the result of not enough blood reaching the head.

Taking a hot shower or sitting in a hot tub immediately after cycling may compound this problem. As your body dissipates heat by increasing its blood flow to the skin, the amount of blood returning to the heart is further compromised. People have been known to faint while taking a hot shower right after cycling.

During cycling the blood vessels of the legs are wide open to carry oxygen and nutrients to your working muscles. The cool-down helps the blood return to your heart by alternately contracting and relaxing the muscles.

What's the Best Cool-Down?

Pedaling slowly in a lower gear (small chainring in front and larger cog in back) provides a pumping action that helps your body's circulation. After a hard cycling session, pedal in this low gear at about 70 to 80 RPM for 4 to 5 minutes. If you have to get off your bicycle, at least keep walking. Continue cycling until your heart rate has returned to below 120 beats per minute.

Stretch after you have cooled down to a heart rate of 120. This is an ideal time for a few additional stretches because your muscles and joints are warm from the cycling. Slow, static stretches will help reduce your muscle soreness. Be sure to pay particular attention to the muscles of the lower back and the legs.

Stretching for Cycling

Experience shows that individuals who are flexible have fewer injuries to the musculoskeletal system. Experts say muscles that are warmed up and then stretched are more efficient and can produce more strength, thus increasing the efficiency of the athlete in an activity.

Relaxed and gentle movements are the most efficient approach to stretching. Each stretch should be gradual, lasting from 20 to 30 seconds. Try to imagine the muscle stretching, the blood pulsing into the muscle area, and the flexibility increasing. Do not rush in anticipation of the workout.

Despite the obvious importance of flexibility, many cyclists often neglect it. They don't stretch before or after they cycle. That is their loss. Increased flexibility won't improve your cardiorespiratory fitness, but it will let you cycle aerobically with greater ease. Flexibility can also reduce your chances of muscle strain and soreness.

The following are some of the most beneficial stretches for cycling. We suggest that you experiment with several of these stretches for about 5 to 8 minutes before and after your ride. The areas of your body that tend to tire first are the ones you should stretch. If you feel tight during the ride, get off your bike and do a few stretches in the areas of your body that seem to be tired and tight. After the ride, stretch those muscle groups that are sore.

Achilles Tendon

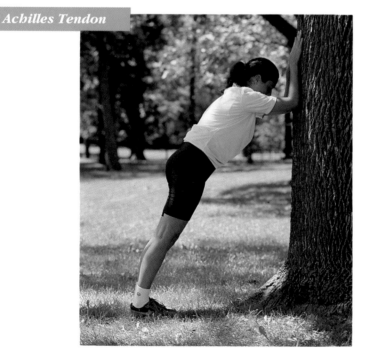

Standing about 2 feet from a vertical surface, place your palms against it, shoulder-width apart and just above your head. Lean forward until your elbows touch the surface, keeping your heels on the ground.

Hamstrings

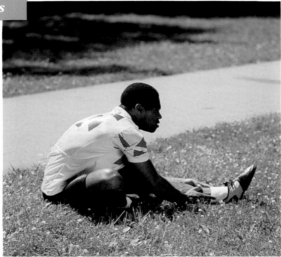

Sit on the ground with both legs extended in front of you. Bend your right knee and slide your heel toward your crotch. Place your heel against the inner side of your left thigh so that a 90-degree angle is formed between the extended leg and the flexed leg. Keeping your left leg straight, bend at the waist, slowly lowering your upper body onto your thigh.

Adductors

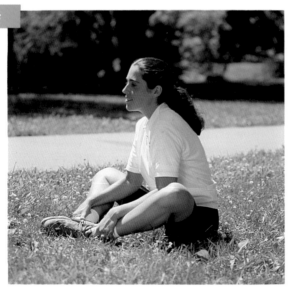

Sit on the ground with your knees bent and the soles of your feet together. Grasp your ankles and lean forward, keeping your back straight as you stretch.

Quadriceps

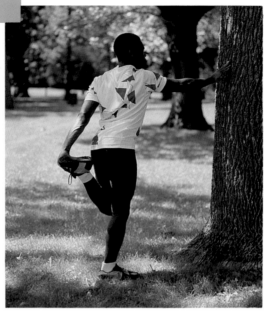

(Don't do this stretch if you have bad knees.) Stand with your right hand against a vertical surface for balance and support. Bend your left leg behind you and grasp the foot with your left hand. Bend your right knee slightly and pull your left heel toward your buttocks. Remember not to overstretch; pull just to the point of tension.

Quadriceps

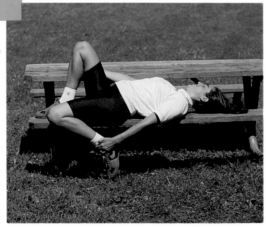

Lie on your back on a table with your left side near the edge. Bend your right leg and slide your foot toward your buttocks; grasp behind your right thigh with your right hand. Lower your left leg off the table and grasp your ankle with your left hand. Slowly pull your left heel toward your buttocks.

Hips

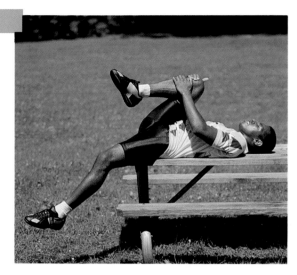

Lie on your back on a table, allowing your left leg to hang over the edge. Bend your right knee, grasp your shin in both hands, and slowly pull your thigh toward your chest.

Buttocks and Hips

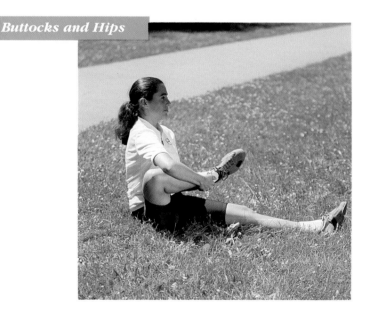

Sit on the floor or ground. Bend your right leg and slide the heel toward you. Grasp the ankle with one hand and hook the knee with your elbow. Pull your foot toward the opposite shoulder.

Lower Back

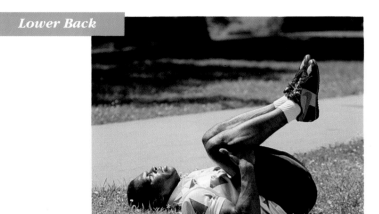

Lying on your back, bend your knees and grasp behind your thighs. Pull your knees toward your chest until your hips come off the ground. Hold for 10 to 20 seconds, then slowly extend one leg, then the other.

Neck

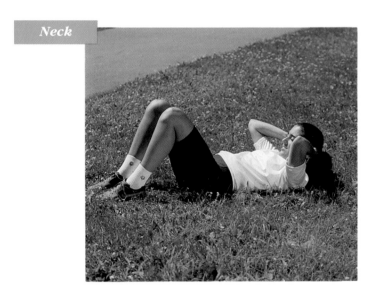

Lie on the ground with both knees bent and your feet on the ground. Lock your hands behind your head and pull your head forward and toward your chest, keeping your shoulder blades on the floor.

Neck

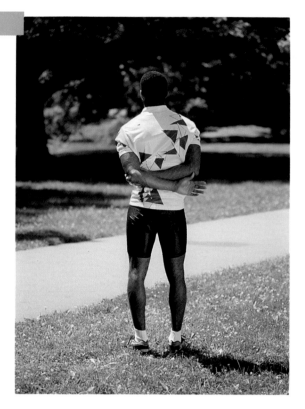

Standing with both arms behind your back, grasp your left elbow from
behind with your right hand. Pull your elbow to the right across your
midline, tilting your head toward your right shoulder (without bending at
the waist).

A proper warm-up increases your metabolism in preparation for faster
and more forceful muscle movements. A cool-down also helps return
blood to the heart to prevent pooling of blood in the legs. Always warm
up before stretching. Always cool down after strenuous cycling, and
include stretching as part of the cool-down regimen.

Now that we have learned the basics of cycling and know our level of
fitness, let's move on to the workout zones.

PART II

CYCLING
WORKOUT ZONES

Workouts in this part of the book are organized into colored zones from lowest to highest intensity—Green, Blue, Purple, Yellow, Orange, and Red. Each zone represents a cluster of workouts that requires you to cycle for a certain period of time within a specified percentage range of your maximum heart rate. Within each zone, the first workout is the least strenuous, the last the most strenuous. Although the zones and the workouts within each zone progress in difficulty, this menu is not designed to move you from one zone to the next as your fitness improves, but rather to provide a variety of cycling workouts that will forestall boredom—the bane of inflexible exercise plans.

Because the intensity of each workout is based on a percentage of your maximum heart rate maintained for a specific period of time, you will use yourself as the standard for picking a zone and a specific exercise within that zone, not some rigid, one-size-fits-all program designed for the "average" cyclist.

The menu of workouts in the following pages provides a wide range of exercise options. The low-intensity zones call for short, relatively easy rides in mostly flat terrain, while the high-intensity zones introduce hill climbing, speedwork, and interval training—a means of improving your fitness more quickly by cycling intensely for a short period, resting, then repeating the effort. Indoor athletes will find a wealth of workouts for stationary bikes, including those that provide upper-body workouts and those that do not. There's a little something for everyone here.

Each workout contains a detailed description of how you are to proceed, including warm-up, stretching, what types of terrain to cover, how briskly to pedal in RPM, approximate distance of the ride, and the number of calories you can expect to burn. The most important items listed in each workout, however, are the percentage of maximum heart rate you'll maintain and how long you'll maintain it—these will tell you how hard you'll have to work.

Your heart rate—not necessarily the distance traveled, the amount of time involved, or the physical workload—tells you the load on your cardiovascular system. In a sense the heart rate pulls all the physiological information together and reports your overall condition with a single number.

Practice taking your pulse to determine your heart rate. This is not difficult, but it usually requires some practice. Your heart rate is recorded in beats per minute. Taking your heart rate manually can only be accomplished safely when you are stopped and have both feet on the ground. Using your index and middle fingers, locate your pulse at the base of your wrist or at the side of your neck. Immediately after you stop cycling, count your heart rate for 15 seconds. Multiply this number by 4 to obtain your heart rate in beats per minute. Again, you may want to consider purchasing a wireless heart monitor to ensure more accuracy when monitoring your heart rate. With such a monitor, you could determine your heart rate without dismounting your bike.

To estimate what your maximum heart rate (max HR) should be, subtract your age from 220 (if you are male) or 226 (if you are female).

Males: max HR = 220 – your age

Females: max HR = 226 – your age.

If you're a 25-year-old male, your heart rate peaks at about 195 beats per minute. If you're a 35-year-old female, it peaks at about 191.

Empirical data leads many fit individuals to question this formula. For example, if you are a 30-year-old female, then your theoretical max HR is 196, but we know one 30-year-old serious female cyclist who has a max HR of 190.

If you use the above formula to determine your max HR, remember that it's only an estimate. The formula will give you a ballpark number to work from, but for a more accurate reading you should consult a physician or an exercise physiologist and have a maximal stress test. For cyclists, this test is usually administered on a bicycle ergometer, which will safely and accurately measure your true maximum heart rate and give you other interesting information, such as your maximum oxygen consumption.

To find the percentage of maximum heart rate you'll be cycling at in each of the workout zones, multiply your max HR by the percent. If you're doing a Green zone workout at 60% of your max HR:

$$\text{max HR} \times .60 = \text{target heart rate.}$$

Another way to estimate effort is simply to ask yourself how you feel. Exercise physiologists have found that your perception of how hard you're working corresponds closely to objective measures such as % max HR. The Rating of Perceived Exertion (RPE) Scale, developed by Dr. Gunnar Borg, will help you estimate how hard you're working. Table II.1 shows how to use the RPE scale to estimate your effort.

Workouts in the Green and Blue zones carry RPE scores of 1 to 3. Purple and Yellow zone workouts carry RPE scores of 4 to 6. Orange and Red zone workouts earn scores of 7 to 9.

Table II.1
Rating of Perceived Exertion (RPE) Scale

1	Very light
2	Light
3	Moderate
4	Somewhat heavy
5	Heavy
6	
7	Very heavy
8	
9	
10	Very, very heavy

Note. From "Psychophysical Bases of Perceived Exertion" by G.A. Borg, 1982, *Medicine and Science in Sports and Exercise*, **14**, pp. 377-387. Copyright 1982 by the American College of Sports Medicine. Adapted by permission.

WORKOUT COLOR ZONES			
Zone (chapter)	Type of workout	RPE	Heart rate
Green (6)	Low intensity, short duration	1-3	60-69%
Blue (7)	Low intensity, long duration	1-3	60-69%
Purple (8)	Medium intensity, short duration	4-6	70-79%
Yellow (9)	Medium intensity, long duration	4-6	70-79%
Orange (10)	High intensity, short duration	7-9	80-89%
Red (11)	High intensity, long duration	7-9	80-89%

Where you start depends on you. If you have little cycling experience or minimal fitness, you might begin with the Green zone workouts. If you are a more advanced cyclist, you may be able to handle workouts like those in the Yellow zone. Ultimately, you'll probably find that blending workouts from different zones is the way to go. To that end, we provide sample programs in Part III. These programs organize the workouts from Part II into a variety of options keyed to your cycling fitness score from chapter 3. They allow you to take advantage of the variety the different zones offer and help you learn how to structure a safe and effective training program.

Vary your workouts. If you feel tired the day after a strenuous Red zone workout, consider doing a low-intensity, short-duration Green zone workout as a recovery ride. Pros and top amateurs call this "active rest," or "resting on the bike." It's a good way to help your body come back from a hard effort. If you feel great the day after a tough Orange zone ride, consider skipping your easy Blue zone spin in favor of a more intense Yellow zone workout. Listen to your body—it's the best personal trainer you could have.

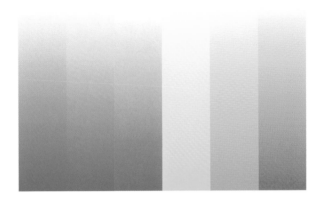

6

Green Zone

The low-intensity, short-duration workouts in the Green zone are intended as introductions to cycling for the newcomer and as recovery rides for the more advanced cyclist. If you're new to cycling, these workouts will help accustom your cardiovascular system to the effort the sport requires and give you a base on which you can construct a more intense exercise program. You might even consider limiting your workouts to the Green zone for a few weeks until you become comfortable on the bike. For more advanced cyclists, a Green zone workout also can help tired muscles recuperate after hard efforts.

In the Green zone, you will be working at 60 to 69% of your maximum heart rate for 20 to 35 minutes. Perceived exertion should be 1 to 3 on the 10-point RPE scale, or light to moderate.

Most of the workouts call for flat roads and steady effort throughout the ride. Shift as necessary to make sure that you're neither bogging down in a gear that's too big or spinning out in one that's too small. The more advanced workouts will have you riding rolling hills—nothing steep, just short, steady climbs—with greater intensity. If your area is short on hills, look for bridges—they almost always have a slight rise to them and will do in a pinch.

On the flats, strive for a pedaling cadence of 85 to 90 RPM (count the number of revolutions one pedal makes in 15 seconds, then multiply the total by 4). While climbing, select a gear in which you can maintain a pedaling cadence of 70 to 80 RPM. This will avoid undue stress on your knees. Upshift or downshift as necessary to maintain the proper cadence.

WORKOUT 1

1

STEADY RIDE
TOTAL TIME: 30 minutes

WARM-UP: 5 minutes easy pedaling in a small gear (90+ RPM)

WORKOUT

Distance: 5 miles
Time: 20 minutes
Terrain: Flat road
Pace: Steady. Shift as needed to keep workload constant. Maintain a cadence of 85-90 RPM.
Effort: 60-65% max HR

COOL-DOWN: 5 minutes easy pedaling in a small gear (85-90+ RPM), then stretching

CALORIES BURNED: About 31 calories per mile

COMMENTS

Concentrate on maintaining the recommended RPM, downshifting or upshifting to keep your workload constant. If you're on a road bike, start to get comfortable with it, moving your hands from the tops of the bars to the brake-lever hoods and onto the "hooks"—the bends in the bars below the brake levers—to minimize discomfort.

WORKOUT 2

STEADY RIDE
TOTAL TIME: 35 minutes

2

WARM-UP: 5 minutes easy pedaling in a small gear (90+ RPM)

WORKOUT

Distance: 6.25 miles

Time: 25 minutes

Terrain: Flat road

Pace: Steady. Shift as needed to keep workload constant. Maintain a cadence of 85-90 RPM.

Effort: 60-65% max HR

COOL-DOWN: 5 minutes easy pedaling in a small gear (85-90+ RPM), then stretching

CALORIES BURNED: About 31 calories per mile

COMMENTS

Maintain the recommended RPM while continuing to become comfortable with your bike. If you have down-tube shifters, practice shifting both levers with one hand. Try removing a water bottle, drinking, and replacing it without looking down.

WORKOUT 3

3

STEADY RIDE
TOTAL TIME: 40 minutes

WARM-UP: 5 minutes easy pedaling in a small gear (90+ RPM)

WORKOUT

Distance: 8 miles

Time: 30 minutes

Terrain: Flat road

Pace: Steady. Shift as necessary to keep workload constant. Maintain a cadence of 85-90 RPM.

Effort: 65-69% max HR

COOL-DOWN: 5 minutes easy pedaling in a small gear (90+ RPM), then stretching

CALORIES BURNED: About 31 calories per mile

COMMENTS

This would make a good midweek ride for the beginner, followed by a day of rest or the shorter Workout 1 as a recovery ride. Practice unwrapping and eating a midride snack without getting off the bike. This is also a good recovery ride for the moderately fit.

WORKOUT 4

STEADY RIDE
TOTAL TIME: 45 minutes

WARM-UP: 5 minutes easy pedaling in a small gear (90+ RPM)

WORKOUT

Distance: 9.5 miles

Time: 35 minutes

Terrain: Flat road

Pace: Steady. Shift as needed to keep workload constant. Maintain a cadence of 85-90 RPM.

Effort: 65-69% max HR

COOL-DOWN: 5 minutes easy pedaling in a small gear (90+ RPM), then stretching

CALORIES BURNED: About 31 calories per mile

COMMENTS

A good midweek ride for beginners or an "active rest" ride for the moderately fit.

WORKOUT 5

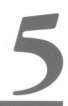

STEADY RIDE
STATIONARY BIKE

TOTAL TIME: 40 minutes

WARM-UP: 5 minutes easy pedaling at zero to light resistance (90+ RPM)

WORKOUT

Time: 30 minutes

Resistance: Light for 15 minutes, then moderate for 15 minutes. Maintain a cadence of 85-90 RPM.

Effort: 60-65% max HR

COOL-DOWN: 5 minutes easy pedaling at zero to light resistance (90+ RPM), then stretching

CALORIES BURNED: About 7-8 calories per minute

COMMENTS

This is a good base-building exercise for beginners and a conditioning-maintenance workout for the moderately fit. Concentrate on maintaining the recommended RPM.

WORKOUT 6

STEADY RIDE
TOTAL TIME: 35 minutes

6

WARM-UP: 10 minutes easy pedaling in a small gear (90+ RPM)

WORKOUT

Distance: 4 miles

Time: 20 minutes

Terrain: Rolling hills

Pace: Steady. Maintain a cadence of 70-80 RPM on hills, 85-90 RPM on flats.

Effort: 65-69% max HR

COOL-DOWN: 5 minutes easy pedaling in a small gear (90+ RPM), then stretching

COMMENTS

This is a shorter ride with a longer warm-up to prepare your legs for the extra stress of hill riding. It also requires attention to cadence; using too big a gear on hills will slow your cadence and can lead to knee problems, so don't hesitate to downshift when necessary. Conversely, upshift on descents to maintain cadence and HR. While climbing, place your hands on the bar tops or the brake hoods and slide back slightly on your saddle for extra leverage.

WORKOUT 7

7

STEADY RIDE
TOTAL TIME: 40 minutes

WARM-UP: 10 minutes easy pedaling in a small gear (90+ RPM)

WORKOUT

Distance: 5 miles
Time: 25 minutes
Terrain: Rolling hills
Pace: Steady. Maintain a cadence of 70-80 RPM on hills, 85-90 RPM on flats.
Effort: 65-69% max HR

COOL-DOWN: 5 minutes easy pedaling in a small gear (90+ RPM), then stretching

CALORIES BURNED: About 31 calories per mile

COMMENTS

Like Green Workout 6, this workout requires a longer warm-up and attention to cadence. Try climbing out of the saddle on steep sections, resting your hands on the brake-lever hoods, and gently rocking the bike from side to side to counterbalance the pumping action of your legs. Shift to a higher gear before standing, then return to a lower gear before sitting.

WORKOUT 8

STEADY RIDE
TOTAL TIME: 45 minutes

8

WARM-UP: 10 minutes easy pedaling in a small gear (90+ RPM)

WORKOUT

Distance: 6 miles

Time: 30 minutes

Terrain: Rolling hills

Pace: Steady. Maintain a cadence of 70-80 RPM on hills, 85-90 RPM on flats.

Effort: 65-69% max HR

COOL-DOWN: 5 minutes easy pedaling in a small gear (90+ RPM), then stretching

CALORIES BURNED: About 31 calories per mile

COMMENTS

This is a good ride for beginners who want to extend their fitness and for moderately fit cyclists who want to maintain their conditioning and plan on riding often in hilly terrain. Upshift and get out of the saddle while cresting hills.

WORKOUT 9

STEADY RIDE
TOTAL TIME: 50 minutes

WARM-UP: 10 minutes easy pedaling in a small gear (90+ RPM)

WORKOUT

Distance: 7 miles

Time: 35 minutes

Terrain: Rolling hills

Pace: Steady. Maintain a cadence of 70-80 RPM on hills, 85-90 RPM on flats.

Effort: 65-69% max HR

COOL-DOWN: 5 minutes easy pedaling in a small gear (90+ RPM), then stretching

CALORIES BURNED: About 31 calories per mile

COMMENTS

A good ride for beginners who want to extend their fitness or for moderately fit cyclists who want to maintain their conditioning. Upshift and get out of the saddle while cresting hills.

WORKOUT 10

STEADY RIDE
STATIONARY BIKE
TOTAL TIME: 45 minutes

10

WARM-UP: 5 minutes easy pedaling at zero to light resistance (90+ RPM)

WORKOUT

Time: 35 minutes

Resistance: Light for 10 minutes, then moderate for 25 minutes. Maintain a cadence of 85-90 RPM.

Effort: 65-69% max HR

COOL-DOWN: 5 minutes easy pedaling at zero to light resistance (90+ RPM), then stretching

CALORIES BURNED: About 7-8 calories per minute

COMMENTS

This is a good base-building exercise for beginners and a maintenance workout for the moderately fit. Concentrate on maintaining the recommended RPM.

		Summary Table		
		Green Zone Workouts		
Workout	**Description**	**Duration**	**Distance**	**Intensity**
1	Steady ride on flat road	20 minutes	5 miles	60-65% max HR
2	Steady ride on flat road	25 minutes	6.25 miles	60-65% max HR
3	Steady ride on flat road	30 minutes	8 miles	65-69% max HR
4	Steady ride on flat road	35 minutes	9.5 miles	65-69% max HR
5	Steady ride at light to moderate intensity	30 minutes	—	60-65% max HR
6	Steady ride on rolling hills	20 minutes	4 miles	65-69% max HR
7	Steady ride on rolling hills	25 minutes	5 miles	65-69% max HR
8	Steady ride on rolling hills	30 minutes	6 miles	65-69% max HR
9	Steady ride on rolling hills	35 minutes	7 miles	65-69% max HR
10	Steady ride at light to moderate intensity	35 minutes	—	65-69% max HR

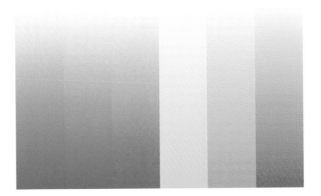

Blue Zone

The long-duration, low-intensity rides in the Blue zone provide additional base fitness work for the newcomer to cycling or other exercise while adding a degree of difficulty not found in the shorter Green zone rides. These rides will help your cardiopulmonary system bring more oxygen to your muscles with fewer respirations, which means you'll be able to breathe easier while riding farther and harder.

In the Blue zone, you will work at 60 to 69% of your maximum heart rate for 30 minutes to an hour. Perceived exertion should be 1 to 3 on the RPE scale, or light to moderate.

Blue zone workouts are good middle-distance efforts, suitable for building a beginner's aerobic strength, for extending a moderately fit cyclist's endurance, or, for the more advanced cyclist, as an active rest day following a short, hard ride, such as those in the Orange zone. Four of the rides require pedaling at a relatively low percentage of your maximum heart rate for a long period, then increasing your intensity slightly for shorter periods. You can do this three ways. You can upshift to a bigger gear, which will build power; you can increase your cadence (RPM), which will build endurance and leg speed; or you can begin your ride on the flats and moving into rolling hills for the intensity work, which will build power and hone your climbing skills. Four of the rides call for sustained climbing at a steady pace; find a long, gradual hill to scale, or a shorter one that can be ridden as part of a loop. If you ride a loop, count only the climbing toward the duration of your workout.

When climbing, pick a gear you can spin at 70 RPM or more and remain seated as much as possible, with your hands on the bar tops or brake-lever hoods; standing brings more muscle groups into play and will quickly drive you beyond your target heart rate. If you decide to stand briefly, either to stretch or to climb a steeper section, upshift to the next smallest cog to keep your workload steady. Gently rock your handlebars from side to side as you climb to balance the thrusting of your legs. Downshift when you resume sitting.

As you venture out for longer periods, you will need to take adequate water and some food to stave off "the bonk," what cyclists call depletion of your body's energy stores. Drink an 8-ounce glass of water before leaving, then drink one bottle of water or sports drink each hour thereafter. Begin to eat lightly—a food bar, banana, or other snack—about 45 minutes into your ride.

If you're using a stationary bike, increase the resistance to simulate hill climbing, then decrease it for the descents. Recover by pedaling easily before increasing the resistance for the next hill.

WORKOUT 1

VARIABLE INTENSITY
TOTAL TIME: 55 minutes

1

WARM-UP: 5 minutes easy pedaling in a small gear (90+ RPM)

WORKOUT

Distance: 12.75 miles

Time: 45 minutes

Terrain: Flat or rolling road

Pace: Variable. Ride 30 minutes at 60-64% of your max HR, then 15 minutes at 65-69% of your max HR. Maintain a cadence of 85-90 RPM.

Effort: 60-69% max HR

COOL-DOWN: 5 minutes easy pedaling in a small gear (90+ RPM), then stretching

CALORIES BURNED: About 31 calories per mile

COMMENTS

A good midweek or end-of-week ride for beginners and a maintenance ride for the moderately fit. Concentrate on your cadence; downshift if it drops during the higher intensity period. Gradual increases in intensity help boost your endurance and average speed.

WORKOUT 2

2

VARIABLE INTENSITY
TOTAL TIME: 1 hour

WARM-UP: 5 minutes easy pedaling in a small gear (90+ RPM)

WORKOUT

Distance: 14 miles

Time: 50 minutes

Terrain: Flat or rolling road

Pace: Variable. Ride 30 minutes at 60-64% of your max HR, then 20 minutes at 65-69% of your max HR. Maintain a cadence of 85-90 RPM.

Effort: 60-69% max HR

COOL-DOWN: 5 minutes easy pedaling in a small gear (90+ RPM), then stretching

CALORIES BURNED: About 31 calories per mile

COMMENTS

A good long ride of the week for beginners or an "active rest" ride for the moderately to highly fit.

WORKOUT 3

VARIABLE INTENSITY
TOTAL TIME: 1 hour 5 minutes

3

WARM-UP: 5 minutes easy pedaling in a small gear (90+ RPM)

WORKOUT

Distance: 15.5 miles
Time: 55 minutes
Terrain: Flat or rolling road
Pace: Variable. Ride 30 minutes at 60-64% of your max HR, then 25 minutes at 65-69% of your max HR. Maintain a cadence of 85-90 RPM.
Effort: 60-69% max HR

COOL-DOWN: 5 minutes easy pedaling in a small gear (90+ RPM), then stretching

CALORIES BURNED: About 31 calories per mile

COMMENTS

A good long ride of the week for beginners or an "active rest" ride for the moderately to highly fit. Try building the intensity gradually—65% of your max HR for 5 minutes, 66% of your max HR for 5 minutes, and so on.

WORKOUT 4

VARIABLE INTENSITY
TOTAL TIME: 1 hour 10 minutes

WARM-UP: 5 minutes easy pedaling in a small gear (90+ RPM)

WORKOUT

Distance: 17 miles

Time: 1 hour

Terrain: Flat or rolling road

Pace: Variable. Ride 30 minutes at 60-64% of your max HR, then 10 minutes at 65-69% of your max HR, followed by 5 minutes at 60-64% of your max HR. Repeat the 10- and 5-minute segments. Maintain a cadence of 85-90 RPM.

Effort: 60-69% max HR

COOL-DOWN: 5 minutes easy pedaling in a small gear (90+ RPM), then stretching

CALORIES BURNED: About 31 calories per mile

COMMENTS

This would make a good midweek ride for a moderately fit cyclist or a long Sunday ride for a beginner. Make the 10-minute intensity sessions as close to 69% of max HR as you can.

WORKOUT 5

VARIABLE RESISTANCE
STATIONARY BIKE

TOTAL TIME: 45 minutes

5

WARM-UP: 10 minutes easy pedaling at zero to light resistance (90+ RPM)

WORKOUT

Time: 30 minutes

Resistance: Light to moderate for "descents," moderate to high for "hills." Increase resistance briefly to simulate hill climbing, recover fully, then increase resistance again. Repeat throughout workout. Maintain a cadence of 70-90 RPM.

Effort: 60% max HR during rest phases, 69% max HR during increased-resistance phases

COOL-DOWN: 5 minutes easy pedaling at light resistance (90+ RPM), then stretching

CALORIES BURNED: About 10-12 calories per minute

COMMENTS

This is a good workout for moderately fit cyclists who want to maintain and improve their conditioning and plan on riding often in hilly terrain.

WORKOUT 6

6

STEADY CLIMB
TOTAL TIME: 45 minutes

WARM-UP: 10 minutes easy pedaling in a small gear (90+ RPM)

WORKOUT

Distance: 5 miles
Time: 30 minutes
Terrain: Gradual hill
Pace: Steady. Maintain a cadence of 70-80 RPM.
Effort: 60-69% max HR

COOL-DOWN: 5 minutes easy pedaling in a small gear (90+ RPM), then stretching

CALORIES BURNED: About 38 calories per mile

COMMENTS

This is a good workout for moderately fit cyclists who want to improve their climbing ability. It's also suitable for beginners who have spent 4 weeks riding flatter terrain. If you can't find a 5-mile hill, find a shorter one and ride as part of a loop, counting only the climbing toward your workout's duration.

WORKOUT 7

STEADY CLIMB
TOTAL TIME: 50 minutes

7

WARM-UP: 10 minutes easy pedaling in a small gear (90+ RPM)

WORKOUT

Distance: 6 miles

Time: 35 minutes

Terrain: Gradual hill

Pace: Steady. Maintain a cadence of 70-80 RPM on hills.

Effort: 60-69% max HR

COOL-DOWN: 5 minutes easy pedaling in a small gear (90+ RPM), then stretching

CALORIES BURNED: About 38 calories per mile

COMMENTS

This is a good midweek workout for moderately fit cyclists and beginners who have spent 4 weeks riding flatter terrain. Stand periodically to bring your upper body into play, remembering to upshift before standing and to downshift before sitting. Your cadence will drop slightly while standing—but if it drops dramatically, you're using too big a gear.

WORKOUT 8

8

STEADY CLIMB
TOTAL TIME: 55 minutes

WARM-UP: 10 minutes easy pedaling in a small gear (90+ RPM)

WORKOUT

Distance: 7 miles
Time: 40 minutes
Terrain: Gradual hill
Pace: Steady. Maintain a cadence of 70-80 RPM.
Effort: 60-69% max HR

COOL-DOWN: 5 minutes easy pedaling in a small gear (90+ RPM), then stretching

CALORIES BURNED: About 38 calories per mile

COMMENTS

Try riding this workout in two ways: first, as a 40-minute sustained climb at 60-64% of your max HR; second, as two 20-minute climbs at 65-69% of your max HR with full recovery between efforts. A good midweek ride for the moderately fit, this could be followed by a rest day or a short-duration, low-intensity ride from the Green zone.

WORKOUT 9

STEADY CLIMB
TOTAL TIME: 1 hour

9

WARM-UP: 10 minutes easy pedaling in a small gear (90+ RPM)

WORKOUT

Distance: 7.75 miles
Time: 45 minutes
Terrain: Gradual hill
Pace: Steady. Maintain a cadence of 70-80 RPM.
Effort: 60-69% max HR

COOL-DOWN: 5 minutes easy pedaling in a small gear (90+ RPM), then stretching

CALORIES BURNED: About 38 calories per mile

COMMENTS

Ride this workout in two ways: first, as a 45-minute sustained climb at 60-64% of your max HR; second, as two 22.5-minute climbs at 65-69% of your max HR with full recovery between efforts. Stand occasionally while climbing, remembering to push a bigger gear while out of the saddle. A good midweek ride for the moderately fit, this could be followed by a rest day or a short-duration, low-intensity ride from the Green zone.

WORKOUT 10

10

VARIABLE RESISTANCE
STATIONARY BIKE
TOTAL TIME: 55 minutes

WARM-UP: 10 minutes easy pedaling at light resistance (90+ RPM)

WORKOUT

Time: 40 minutes

Resistance: Light to moderate for "descents," moderate to high for "hills." Increase resistance briefly to simulate hill climbing, recover fully, then increase resistance again. Repeat throughout workout. Maintain a cadence of 70-90 RPM.

Effort: 60% of max HR during rest phases, 69% of max HR during increased-resistance phases

COOL-DOWN: 5 minutes easy pedaling at light resistance (90+ RPM), then stretching

CALORIES BURNED: About 10-12 calories per minute

COMMENTS

This is a good workout for moderately fit cyclists who want to maintain and improve their conditioning and who plan on riding often in hilly terrain.

Summary Table
Blue Zone Workouts

Workout	Description	Duration	Distance	Intensity
1	Variable intensity on flat or rolling road	45 minutes	12.75 miles	60-69% max HR
2	Variable intensity on flat or rolling road	50 minutes	14 miles	60-69% max HR
3	Variable intensity on flat or rolling road	55 minutes	15.5 miles	60-69% max HR
4	Variable intensity on flat or rolling road	1 hour	17 miles	60-69% max HR
5	Variable intensity	30 minutes	—	60-69% max HR
6	Steady climb on gradual hill	30 minutes	5 miles	60-69% max HR
7	Steady climb on gradual hill	35 minutes	6 miles	60-69% max HR
8	Steady climb on gradual hill	40 minutes	7 miles	60-69% max HR
9	Steady climb on gradual hill	45 minutes	7.75 miles	60-69% max HR
10	Variable intensity	40 minutes	—	60-69% max HR

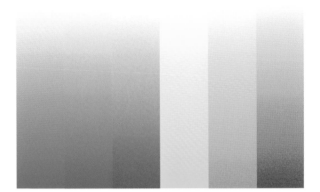

8

Purple Zone

The medium-intensity, short-duration Purple zone workouts are more strenuous than those in the Green or Blue zones—and since you'll be riding harder, you'll be logging fewer miles and minutes. Heart rates range from 70 to 79% of your maximum, and duration varies from 20 to 50 minutes. Perceived exertion should be 4 to 6 on the RPE scale, or somewhat heavy to heavy.

The Purple zone's hill workouts will further expand your aerobic power and muscular strength, bringing upper-body muscle groups into play as you pull on the handlebars to augment the power of your legs. In some respects, it resembles a weightlifting workout using heavy weights with low repetitions—your pedaling cadence, or reps, will be considerably slower than on the flats, while gravity provides the weights.

The upper-body workout involved in hill climbing on the road or trail can be mimicked to some degree by stationary bikes with levers that involve the arms. If yours doesn't have such a setup, simply increase the resistance to simulate climbing, then pull rhythmically on the handlebars in concert with your pedal strokes. Make sure you don't bog down in your cadence, maintaining at least 70 RPM while "climbing."

Purple zone workouts make good early week rides for beginners or midweek rides for moderately fit cyclists and highly fit cyclists; they also make good pre-event tune-ups for competitors. If you have not ridden any hills, consider beginning with some Blue zone work before venturing into the hilly portion of the Purple zone. Extended climbs are hard on the knees and lower back, so it's best to begin gradually.

The rolling-road and flat-road workouts call for a variable pace, alternating periods of greater and lesser intensity. If you're riding a road bike, move your hands to the dropped portion of the handlebars for the work phases, then return to the brake-lever hoods or bar tops for the rest phases. Maintain the recommended heart rates and cadences, shifting as necessary.

Some Purple zone workouts call for you to create a loop that can be ridden more than once; try to find one with little or no traffic that's free of stop signs and traffic lights. Shopping malls or office parks after hours, parks closed to auto traffic, and housing developments under construction make excellent courses. Where possible, create loops with both left- and right-hand corners to give you experience in turning in both directions.

WORKOUT 1

STEADY CLIMB
TOTAL TIME: 35 minutes

1

WARM-UP: 10 minutes easy pedaling in a small gear (90+ RPM)

WORKOUT

Distance: 4 miles

Time: 20 minutes

Terrain: Long, gradual hill

Pace: Steady. Maintain a cadence of 75-80 RPM.

COOL-DOWN: 5 minutes easy pedaling in a small gear (90+ RPM), then stretching

CALORIES BURNED: About 47 calories per mile

COMMENTS

A good workout for beginners and moderately fit cyclists who want to improve their power and climbing ability. Highly fit cyclists can repeat the whole workout 1 or more times at the upper end of the max HR range, making sure to recover fully between climbs.

WORKOUT 2

2

VARIABLE INTENSITY CLIMB
TOTAL TIME: 35 minutes

WARM-UP: 10 minutes easy pedaling in a small gear (90+ RPM)

WORKOUT

Distance: 4.5 miles

Time: 20 minutes

Terrain: Long, gradual hill

Pace: Variable. Climb 10 minutes at 75-79% of your max HR, then shift into a lower gear to recover fully at 70-74% of your max HR. Perform this sequence twice. Maintain a cadence of 75-80 RPM.

Effort: 70-79% max HR

COOL-DOWN: 5 minutes easy pedaling in a small gear (90+ RPM), then stretching

CALORIES BURNED: About 47 calories per mile

COMMENTS

Good for beginners and moderately fit cyclists who want to improve their climbing. Maintain the recommended HR during all phases, shifting as necessary. Recover fully between 10-minute efforts. Highly fit cyclists can repeat the workout 1 or more times.

WORKOUT 3

VARIABLE INTENSITY CLIMB
TOTAL TIME: 35 minutes

3

WARM-UP: 10 minutes easy pedaling in a small gear (90+ RPM)

WORKOUT

Distance: 4.5 miles

Time: 20 minutes

Terrain: Loop with a 5-minute climb

Pace: Variable. Climb 5 minutes at 79% of your max HR, then recover at 70% of your max HR. Perform this climb and recovery 4 times. Maintain a cadence of 75-80 RPM.

Effort: 70-79% max HR

COOL-DOWN: 5 minutes easy pedaling in a small gear (90+ RPM), then stretching

CALORIES BURNED: About 47 calories per mile

COMMENTS

A good workout for moderately fit cyclists who want to improve their power and climbing ability. Maintain the recommended HR during all phases, shifting as necessary. Upshift and get out of the saddle as you crest the hill—this will help you build power and acceleration. Highly fit cyclists can repeat the workout 1 or more times.

WORKOUT 4

VARIABLE INTENSITY CLIMB
TOTAL TIME: 40 minutes

WARM-UP: 10 minutes easy pedaling in a small gear (90+ RPM)

WORKOUT

Distance: 5 miles

Time: 25 minutes

Terrain: Loop with a 5-minute climb

Pace: Variable. Ride 5 minutes at 79% of your max HR, then recover at 70% of your max HR. Perform this climb and recovery 5 times. Maintain a cadence of 75-80 RPM.

Effort: 70-79% max HR

COOL-DOWN: 5 minutes easy pedaling in a small gear (90+ RPM), then stretching

CALORIES BURNED: About 47 calories per mile

COMMENTS

This is a good workout for moderately fit cyclists who want to improve their climbing ability. Maintain the recommended HR during all phases, shifting as necessary. Upshift and get out of the saddle as you crest the hill—this will help you build power and acceleration. Highly fit cyclists can repeat the workout 1 or more times.

WORKOUT 5

STEADY RIDE
STATIONARY BIKE

TOTAL TIME: 45 minutes

WARM-UP: 10 minutes easy pedaling at light resistance (90+ RPM)

WORKOUT

Time: 30 minutes

Resistance: Moderate to high. Maintain a cadence of 75-80 RPM.

Effort: 70-74% max HR

COOL-DOWN: 5 minutes easy pedaling at light resistance (90+ RPM), then stretching

CALORIES BURNED: About 13-15 calories per minute

COMMENTS

This is a good workout for moderately fit cyclists who want to improve their climbing or their ability to cycle at high intensity for longer periods of time.

WORKOUT 6

6

TIME TRIAL
TOTAL TIME: 45 minutes

WARM-UP: 10 minutes easy pedaling in a small gear (90+ RPM)

WORKOUT

Distance: 8.5 miles
Time: 30 minutes
Terrain: Rolling road
Pace: Fast. Maintain a cadence of 90+ RPM.
Effort: 70-74% max HR on flats, 75-79% max HR
   on hills

COOL-DOWN: 5 minutes easy pedaling in a small gear (90+ RPM), then stretching

CALORIES BURNED: About 47 calories per mile

COMMENTS

This is a good midweek workout for beginners and moderately fit cyclists who want to improve their ability to cycle more intensely for short periods. Pick a route that takes longer than 30 minutes to ride—preferably one without stop signs or traffic lights—then strive to increase your speed with weekly rides on the same route. Achieve this either by raising your cadence or upshifting, until you can ride it in a half hour or less. The first builds speed; the second, power. Keep track of your times to chart your improvement.

WORKOUT 7

SPEEDWORK
TOTAL TIME: 55 minutes

7

WARM-UP: 10 minutes easy pedaling in a small gear (90+ RPM)

WORKOUT

Distance: 10-12 miles

Time: 40 minutes

Terrain: Flat to rolling 1-mile circuit

Pace: Fast. Ride 1 lap hard, then 1 lap recovery in a smaller gear. Perform this sequence 5 times. Maintain a cadence of 90 RPM.

Effort: 75-79% max HR during work, 70-74% max HR during rest

COOL-DOWN: 5 minutes easy pedaling in a small gear (90+ RPM), then stretching

CALORIES BURNED: About 47 calories per mile

COMMENTS

Create your 1-mile course in a low-traffic housing development, an industrial/office park after business hours, or a park, using both left- and right-hand turns if possible. Maintain the recommended cadence, shifting as necessary to keep your HR within the prescribed ranges. This is a good workout for moderately fit cyclists who want to improve their ability to cycle intensely for short periods or for highly fit cyclists who want a pre-event tune-up.

WORKOUT 8

SPEEDWORK
TOTAL TIME: 55 minutes

WARM-UP: 10 minutes easy pedaling in a small gear (90+ RPM)

WORKOUT

Distance: 10 miles

Time: 40 minutes

Terrain: Flat to rolling road

Pace: Fast. Ride 5 minutes at 75-79% of your max HR, then 5 minutes at 70-74% of your max HR. Perform this sequence 4 times. Maintain a cadence of 90 RPM.

Effort: 70-79% max HR

COOL-DOWN: 5 minutes easy pedaling in a small gear (90+ RPM), then stretching

CALORIES BURNED: About 47 calories per mile

COMMENTS

Maintain the recommended cadence, shifting as necessary to keep your HR within the prescribed ranges. A good workout for moderately fit cyclists who want to improve their ability to cycle intensely for short periods or for beginners who want to extend their endurance.

SPEEDWORK
TOTAL TIME: 1 hour 5 minutes

2

WARM-UP: 10 minutes easy pedaling in a small gear (90+ RPM)

WORKOUT

Distance: 12 miles

Time: 50 minutes

Terrain: Flat to rolling road

Pace: Fast. Ride 5 minutes at 75-79% of your max HR, then 5 minutes at 70-74% of your max HR. Perform this sequence 5 times. Maintain a cadence of 90 RPM.

Effort: 70-79% max HR

COOL-DOWN: 5 minutes easy pedaling in a small gear (90+ RPM), then stretching

CALORIES BURNED: About 47 calories per mile

COMMENTS

Maintain the recommended cadence, shifting as necessary to keep your HR within the prescribed ranges. A good workout for moderately fit cyclists who want to improve their ability to cycle intensely for short periods or for beginners who want to extend their endurance.

WORKOUT 10

10

STEADY RIDE
STATIONARY BIKE

TOTAL TIME: 1 hour

WARM-UP: 10 minutes easy pedaling at light resistance (90+ RPM)

WORKOUT

Time: 45 minutes

Resistance: Brisk, steady effort at moderate resistance. Maintain a cadence of 90-100 RPM.

Effort: 75-79% max HR

COOL-DOWN: 5 minutes easy pedaling at light resistance (90+ RPM), then stretching

CALORIES BURNED: About 13-15 calories per minute

COMMENTS

This is a good workout for moderately fit cyclists who want to improve their speed and their ability to cycle hard for extended periods.

	Summary Table Purple Zone Workouts			
Workout	**Description**	**Duration**	**Distance**	**Intensity**
1	Steady climb on long, gradual hill	20 minutes	4 miles	70-79% max HR
2	Variable intensity climb on long, gradual hill	20 minutes	4.5 miles	70-79% max HR
3	Variable intensity climb	20 minutes	4.5 miles	70-79% max HR
4	Variable intensity climb	25 minutes	5 miles	70-79% max HR
5	Variable intensity	30 minutes	—	70-74% max HR
6	Time trial on rolling road	30 minutes	8.5 miles	70-79% max HR
7	Speedwork on flat to rolling 1-mile circuit	40 minutes	10-12 miles	70-79% max HR
8	Speedwork on flat to rolling road	40 minutes	10 miles	70-79% max HR
9	Speedwork on flat to rolling road	50 minutes	12 miles	70-79% max HR
10	Steady ride at moderate intensity	45 minutes	—	75-79% max HR

9

Yellow Zone

Yellow zone workouts are medium-intensity, long-duration efforts. Heart rates range from 70 to 79% of your maximum, and duration ranges from 30 minutes to 1 hour 15 minutes. Perceived exertion should be 4 to 6 on the RPE scale, or somewhat heavy to heavy.

The best way to add intensity to a cycling program is to ride hills; they force you to work harder without the regimentation of a timed interval workout. Be certain you have a good base—4 weeks or more of flatland or rolling-hill riding—before hitting the big hills.

If your area is short on places to climb, aerobic intervals are a good substitute. In interval training, you will ride at high intensity for a period, then rest for a period 2 to 3 times as long, then repeat the work/rest intervals a number of times. Don't quit pedaling during the rest periods—continue to pedal, but in a smaller gear. Aerobic intervals are good training for competitors—triathletes, time trialists, road racers—and for casual riders, too. They increase aerobic power, endurance, and muscle strength.

Moderately fit cyclists might do their intervals at midweek, on the flats. Highly fit cyclists can blend aerobic intervals and hills for an extra-intense workout that's good for a midweek or Saturday ride. If your friends fly away from you on hills, hill intervals can give you the power and endurance you need to keep up with them. If you're interested in competition, this will give you some feel for the changes in tempo that are common in racing. Newcomers to cycling or serious exercise should build an aerobic base with workouts from the Green, Blue, or Purple zones before attempting a Yellow zone session.

WORKOUT 1

1

AEROBIC INTERVALS

TOTAL TIME: 1 hour 15 minutes

WARM-UP: 10 minutes easy pedaling in a small gear (90+ RPM)

WORKOUT

Distance: 17-19 miles

Time: 1 hour

Terrain: Rolling hills

Pace: Variable. Ride 5 minutes at 75-79% of your max HR, then 10 minutes at 70-74% of your max HR. Perform this sequence 4 times. Maintain a cadence of 75-90 RPM.

Effort: 70-79% max HR

COOL-DOWN: 5 minutes easy pedaling in a small gear (90+ RPM), then stretching

CALORIES BURNED: About 47 calories per mile

COMMENTS

Good for moderately and highly fit cyclists who want to improve their endurance. Maintain the recommended HR and cadence during all phases, shifting as necessary. Highly fit cyclists can repeat the workout 1 or more times.

WORKOUT 2

AEROBIC INTERVALS
TOTAL TIME: 1 hour 30 minutes

WARM-UP: 10 minutes easy pedaling in a small gear (90+ RPM)

WORKOUT

Distance: 20-22 miles

Time: 1 hour 15 minutes

Terrain: Rolling hills

Pace: Variable. Ride 5 minutes at 75-79% of your max HR, then 10 minutes at 70-74% of your max HR. Perform this sequence 5 times. Maintain a cadence of 75-90 RPM.

Effort: 70-79% max HR

COOL-DOWN: 5 minutes easy pedaling in a small gear (90+ RPM), then stretching

CALORIES BURNED: About 47 calories per mile

COMMENTS

Good for moderately and highly fit cyclists who want to improve their endurance. Maintain the recommended HR and cadence during all phases, shifting as necessary. Highly fit cyclists can repeat the workout 1 or more times.

WORKOUT 3

3

AEROBIC INTERVALS/
VARIABLE INTENSITY CLIMB
TOTAL TIME: 1 hour 15 minutes

WARM-UP: 10 minutes easy pedaling in a small gear (90+ RPM)

WORKOUT

Distance: 13-15 miles

Time: 1 hour

Terrain: Long, gradual hill

Pace: Variable. Ride 5 minutes at 75-79% of your max HR, then 10 minutes at 70-74% of your max HR. Perform this sequence 4 times. Maintain a cadence of 75-90 RPM.

Effort: 70-79% max HR

COOL-DOWN: 5 minutes easy pedaling in a small gear (90+ RPM), then stretching

CALORIES BURNED: About 47 calories per mile

COMMENTS

Good for moderately and highly fit cyclists who want to improve their power and climbing. Maintain the recommended HR and cadence during all phases, shifting as necessary. If you can't find an hour-long hill, ride a shorter one as part of a loop, counting only the climbing toward your time. Highly fit cyclists can repeat the workout 1 or more times.

WORKOUT 4

AEROBIC INTERVALS/
VARIABLE INTENSITY CLIMB

TOTAL TIME: 1 hour 30 minutes

WARM-UP: 10 minutes easy pedaling in a small gear (90+ RPM)

WORKOUT

Distance: 15-17 miles

Time: 1 hour 15 minutes

Terrain: Long, gradual hill

Pace: Variable. Ride 5 minutes at 75-79% of your max HR, then 10 minutes at 70-74% of your max HR. Perform this sequence 5 times. Maintain a cadence of 75-90 RPM.

Effort: 70-79% max HR

COOL-DOWN: 5 minutes easy pedaling in a small gear (90+ RPM), then stretching

CALORIES BURNED: About 47 calories per mile

COMMENTS

Good for moderately and highly fit cyclists who want to improve their power and climbing. Maintain the recommended HR and cadence during all phases, shifting as necessary. If you can't find an hour-long hill, ride a shorter one as part of a loop, counting only the climbing toward your duration. Highly fit cyclists can repeat the workout 1 or more times.

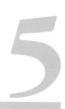

VARIABLE INTENSITY
STATIONARY BIKE

TIME: 1 hour

WARM-UP: 10 minutes easy pedaling at light resistance (90+ RPM)

WORKOUT

Time: 45 minutes

Resistance: Moderate to high. Ride hard for 5 minutes, then recover for 10 minutes. Perform this sequence 3 times. Maintain a cadence of 90-100 RPM.

Effort: 75-79% max HR

COOL-DOWN: 5 minutes easy pedaling at light resistance (90+ RPM), then stretching

CALORIES BURNED: About 13-15 calories per minute

COMMENTS

Good for cyclists who need to increase their power and their ability to cycle hard for extended periods. To stay motivated during long indoor workouts, set up your bike in front of a TV and watch cycling tapes, record a 45-minute medley of motivational music to listen to while you ride, or mix the two. (Be careful that your cadence does not rise or fall erratically in time with the music.)

WORKOUT 6

AEROBIC INTERVALS
TOTAL TIME: 1 hour 15 minutes

WARM-UP: 10 minutes easy pedaling in a small gear (90+ RPM)

WORKOUT

Distance: 17-19 miles

Time: 1 hour

Terrain: Flat

Pace: Variable. Ride 5 minutes at 75-79% of your max HR, then 10 minutes at 70-74% of your max HR. Perform this sequence 4 times. Maintain a cadence of 110+ RPM during work, 90 RPM during rest.

Effort: 70-79% max HR

COOL-DOWN: 5 minutes easy pedaling in a small gear (90+ RPM), then stretching

CALORIES BURNED: About 47 calories per mile

COMMENTS

Upshifting to achieve your target HR during the work phase will help you build power. Increasing your pedaling cadence will help you build leg speed. Both are useful in a variety of cycling situations, from racing to getting through busy intersections to beating a rainstorm home.

7 AEROBIC INTERVALS

TOTAL TIME: 1 hour 30 minutes

WARM-UP: 10 minutes easy pedaling in a small gear (90+ RPM)

WORKOUT

Distance: 20-22 miles

Time: 1 hour 15 minutes

Terrain: Flat

Pace: Variable. Ride 5 minutes at 75-79% of your max HR, then 10 minutes at 70-74% of your max HR. Perform this sequence 5 times. Maintain a cadence of 110+ RPM during work, 90 RPM during rest.

Effort: 70-79% max HR

COOL-DOWN: 5 minutes easy pedaling in a small gear (90+ RPM), then stretching

CALORIES BURNED: About 47 calories per mile

COMMENTS

Upshifting during the work phase builds power; increasing your pedaling cadence builds leg speed.

WORKOUT 8

AEROBIC INTERVALS
TOTAL TIME: 1 hour 15 minutes

8

WARM-UP: 10 minutes easy pedaling in a small gear (90+ RPM)

WORKOUT

Distance: 17-19 miles

Time: 1 hour

Terrain: Rolling hills

Pace: Variable. Ride 5 minutes at 75-79% of your max HR, then 10 minutes at 70-74% of your max HR. Perform this sequence 4 times. Maintain a cadence of 80-110+ RPM.

Effort: 70-79% max HR

COOL-DOWN: 5 minutes easy pedaling in a small gear (90+ RPM), then stretching

CALORIES BURNED: About 47 calories per mile

COMMENTS

This adds a wild card to your training. Some work phases will come up on hills, others on descents. Strive for a smooth pedal stroke, neither bogging down on climbs nor spinning out on descents, shifting as necessary.

WORKOUT 9

AEROBIC INTERVALS
TOTAL TIME: 1 hour 30 minutes

WARM-UP: 10 minutes easy pedaling in a small gear (90+ RPM)

WORKOUT

Distance: 20-22 miles

Time: 1 hour 15 minutes

Terrain: Flat

Pace: Variable. Ride 5 minutes at 75-79% of your max HR, then 10 minutes at 70-74% of your max HR. Perform this sequence 5 times. Maintain a cadence of 110+ RPM during work, 90 RPM during rest.

Effort: 70-79% max HR

COOL-DOWN: 5 minutes easy pedaling in a small gear (90+ RPM), then stretching

CALORIES BURNED: About 47 calories per mile

COMMENTS

Instead of upshifting to achieve your target HR during the work phase, increase your pedaling cadence. On climbs, this will build power; on flats and descents, it will build speed.

WORKOUT 10

TIME TRIAL
STATIONARY BIKE

TOTAL TIME: 50 minutes

WARM-UP: 15 minutes spinning (90+ RPM), increasing resistance every 5 minutes

WORKOUT

Time: 30 minutes

Resistance: Moderate to high. Ride at 75-79% of your max HR for 30 minutes. Maintain a cadence of 90+ RPM.

Effort: 75-79% max HR

COOL-DOWN: 5 minutes easy pedaling at light resistance (90+ RPM), then stretching

CALORIES BURNED: About 13-15 calories per minute

COMMENTS

Good for cyclists who need to increase their power and their ability to cycle hard for extended periods.

Workout	Description	Duration	Distance	Intensity
1	Aerobic intervals on rolling hills	1 hour	17-19 miles	70-79% max HR
2	Aerobic intervals on rolling hills	1 hour 15 minutes	20-22 miles	70-79% max HR
3	Aerobic intervals on long, gradual hill	1 hour	13-15 miles	70-79% max HR
4	Aerobic intervals on long, gradual hill	1 hour 15 minutes	15-17 miles	70-79% max HR
5	Variable intensity	45 minutes	—	75-79% max HR
6	Aerobic intervals on flat terrain	1 hour	17-19 miles	70-79% max HR
7	Aerobic intervals on flat terrain	1 hour 15 minutes	20-22 miles	70-79% max HR
8	Aerobic intervals on rolling hills	1 hour	17-19 miles	70-79% max HR
9	Aerobic intervals on flat terrain	1 hour 15 minutes	20-22 miles	70-79% max HR
10	Time trial at moderate to high intensity	30 minutes	—	75-79% max HR

10

Orange Zone

Anaerobic threshold training comes into play in the Orange zone. Workouts in this zone last for a short period (10 to 30 minutes), but they require you to work at high intensity (80 to 90% of your maximum heart rate) during the work portions. Perceived exertion on the RPE scale should be 7+, or very heavy.

Intervals at this level of exertion constitute anaerobic threshold training, which increases your body's ability to take in oxygen quicker than simply riding long distances at low intensity. It requires you to ride hard for a short period, rest 3 times longer than that period, then ride hard again, repeating the on/off intervals a set number of times. Working at above-normal intensity for short periods will help you ride harder and faster for longer periods. If you are new to cycling or beginning your first serious exercise program, build an aerobic base with workouts from the Green, Blue, Purple, or Yellow zones before attempting an Orange zone session.

Always warm up for 10 to 15 minutes by riding easily in a small gear before attempting an interval workout. Similarly, cool down afterward. When beginning the work period, upshift, come up out of the saddle, and accelerate smoothly; then sit for the remainder of the interval—you want to achieve your target heart rate as quickly as possible. During the rest periods, don't quit pedaling—spin at high RPM, but in a smaller gear. And begin your interval training on flat terrain—hill intervals are among the hardest workouts in a racer's repertoire.

On a stationary bike, increase resistance for the work phase, then decrease it for the off phase. Make certain you don't bog down against the increased resistance, maintaining a pedaling cadence of at least 80 RPM. If you don't like riding indoors, these are good workouts for you. They require minimal time but return maximal results.

Orange zone workouts can be used in a number of different ways. Their intensity makes them a good way to begin your week after a day of rest. You may add an Orange zone interval workout to your weekly schedule (1 or 2 a week is plenty, with at least 1 easier day in between efforts). You can use a comparatively easy Green zone workout as a warm-up for a more intense Orange zone workout. Or you may treat an Orange zone workout as a single set in a multiple-set workout. If you decide on a multiple-set workout, be sure to recover completely between sets, letting your heart rate drop to at least 130 beats per minute before beginning your next set.

You can also work on biomechanical deficiencies during an interval session. If you have trouble maintaining a 90 RPM cadence, do your intervals in a small gear—this requires you to pedal quickly and smoothly if you are to maintain the required heart rate. If you lack the strength necessary to ride in a big gear, or you want to build leg power for climbing, do your intervals in a big gear at a lower cadence, say 70 to 80 RPM.

When doing sprints, avoid using a gear that's too big for you. Instead, select a gear that takes some effort to get rolling, but one that you can spin out in 20 seconds or so without bouncing up and down on the saddle. This will build both power and leg speed, both essential components of sprinting. Let your legs and lungs be your guide. It's tempting to think that a big gear equals big speed, but it can lead to injury.

In time trials, choose a gear you think you can push for the distance and maintain a steady pace, shifting only when necessary to maintain your cadence and workload. Avoid sudden decelerations and accelerations— they'll wear you out faster than a smooth, sustained effort.

WORKOUT 1

INTERVALS
TOTAL TIME: 35 minutes

WARM-UP: 15 minutes spinning at 90 RPM, gradually increasing the gear

WORKOUT

Distance: 3.5 miles
Time: 10 minutes
Terrain: Flat road
Pace: Variable. Ride 30 seconds at 80-90% max HR, then rest for 90 seconds at about 75% max HR. Perform this sequence 5 times. Maintain a cadence of 90-100 RPM during work phase.
Effort: 75-90% max HR

COOL-DOWN: 10 minutes easy pedaling in a small gear (90+ RPM), then stretching

CALORIES BURNED: About 55 calories per mile

COMMENTS

This is a good workout for moderately fit cyclists who want to improve their speed, acceleration, and ability to cycle intensely or for highly fit cyclists who want a preevent tune-up. Done in sets of 5 to 7 repetitions, with full recovery between sets, this is also a good workout for the highly fit. Add sets gradually.

WORKOUT 2

2

INTERVALS

TOTAL TIME: 35 minutes

WARM-UP: 15 minutes spinning at 90 RPM, gradually increasing the gear

WORKOUT

Distance: 2.5 miles
Time: 10 minutes
Terrain: Rolling hills
Pace: Variable. Ride 30 seconds at 85-90% max HR, then rest for 90 seconds at about 75% max HR. Perform this sequence 5 times. Maintain a cadence of 80-90 RPM.
Effort: 75-90% max HR

COOL-DOWN: 10 minutes easy pedaling in a small gear (90+ RPM), then stretching

CALORIES BURNED: About 55 calories per mile

COMMENTS

This is a good workout for moderately fit cyclists who want to improve their speed, power, and ability to cycle intensely. Work phases that coincide with climbs will build power, whereas those done on descents will build speed and fluidity in pedal stroke. Done in sets of 5 to 7 repetitions, with full recovery between sets, this is also a good workout for the highly fit. Add sets gradually.

WORKOUT 3

INTERVALS
TOTAL TIME: 35 minutes

3

WARM-UP: 15 minutes spinning at 90 RPM, gradually increasing the gear

WORKOUT

Distance: 2 miles
Time: 10 minutes
Terrain: Extended climb
Pace: Variable. Ride 30 seconds at 90% max HR, then rest for 90 seconds at about 75% max HR. Perform this sequence 5 times. Maintain a cadence of 70-90 RPM.
Effort: 75-90% max HR

COOL-DOWN: 10 minutes easy pedaling in a small gear (90+ RPM), then stretching

CALORIES BURNED: About 55 calories per mile

COMMENTS

This is a good workout for moderately fit cyclists who want to improve their power and ability to cycle intensely. Done in sets of 5 to 7 repetitions, with full recovery between sets, it is also a good workout for the highly fit. Add sets gradually.

WORKOUT 4

SPEEDPLAY
TOTAL TIME: 55 minutes

WARM-UP: 15 minutes spinning at 90 RPM, gradually increasing the gear

WORKOUT

Distance: 9-11 miles
Time: 30 minutes
Terrain: Flat to rolling hills
Pace: Fast. Random, all-out accelerations (20+ seconds). Maintain a cadence of 80-100 RPM.
Effort: 90% max HR during work phase

COOL-DOWN: 10 minutes easy pedaling in a small gear (90+ RPM), then stretching

CALORIES BURNED: About 55 calories per mile

COMMENTS

Moderately and highly fit cyclists who want to improve their acceleration and speed will find this workout both useful and entertaining. It's best done in a group, with several people deciding when to "hammer." Accelerating on descents will build your leg speed, while jumping on hills will build power and "snap."

WORKOUT 5

INTERVALS
STATIONARY BIKE

TOTAL TIME: 50 minutes

WARM-UP: 15 minutes at 90+ RPM—5 minutes at zero resistance, 5 minutes at light resistance, 5 minutes at moderate resistance

WORKOUT

Time: 30 minutes

Resistance: Moderate to high during work intervals, light during rest. Ride 30 seconds at 85-90% max HR, then rest for 90 seconds at about 75% max HR. Perform this sequence 5 times. Do 3 sets with full recovery between each. Maintain a cadence of 90-100 RPM.

Effort: 75-90% max HR

COOL-DOWN: 5 minutes easy pedaling at light resistance (90+ RPM), then stretching

CALORIES BURNED: About 13-15 calories per minute during high intensity phases

COMMENTS

This is a good workout for highly and moderately fit cyclists who want to improve their ability to cycle intensely. Done at high resistance, it can increase power; at moderate to low resistance, it can increase pedal cadence and speed.

WORKOUT 6

6

TIME TRIAL
TOTAL TIME: 1 hour 10 minutes

WARM-UP: 30 minutes spinning at 90 RPM, gradually increasing size of the gear

WORKOUT

Distance: 10 miles

Time: 30 minutes

Terrain: Flat to rolling hills

Pace: Fast. Select a 10-mile course with no stop signs or traffic lights and maintain a cadence of 90+ RPM.

Effort: 80-90% max HR

COOL-DOWN: 10 minutes easy pedaling in a small gear (90+ RPM), then stretching

CALORIES BURNED: About 47 calories per mile

COMMENTS

This is a great fitness indicator for moderately and highly fit cyclists who are considering competition. It also adds some spice to the workout routine, particularly when done with friends. Try to maintain the recommended RPM and HR throughout the ride. Note your time, then repeat the workout weekly (perhaps on Saturday) to gauge improvement. A consistent failure to improve your time may indicate overtraining or illness.

WORKOUT 7

TIME TRIAL

TOTAL TIME: 1 hour 10 minutes

WARM-UP: 30 minutes spinning at 90 RPM, gradually increasing size of the gear

WORKOUT

Distance: 5 miles

Time: 30± minutes

Terrain: Long, moderately steep hill

Pace: Fast. Select a 5-mile climb with no stop signs or traffic lights and maintain a cadence of 90+ RPM.

Effort: 80-90% max HR

COOL-DOWN: 10 minutes easy pedaling in a small gear (90+ RPM), then stretching

CALORIES BURNED: About 47 calories per mile

COMMENTS

This is a great power-builder and fitness indicator for moderately and highly fit cyclists who are considering competition. It is particularly enjoyable when done with friends. Try to maintain the recommended RPM and HR throughout the ride. Note your time, then repeat the workout weekly (perhaps on Saturday) to gauge improvement. A consistent failure to improve your time may indicate overtraining or illness.

WORKOUT 8

8 VARIABLE INTENSITY CLIMB
TOTAL TIME: 45 minutes

WARM-UP: 10 minutes easy pedaling in small gear (90+ RPM)

WORKOUT

Distance: 7-9 miles

Time: 30 minutes

Terrain: 2-mile loop with several short, steep hills

Pace: Variable. Ride hard on climbs, rest on descents and flats. Maintain a cadence of 75-80 RPM.

Effort: 85-90% max HR during work phase

COOL-DOWN: 5 minutes easy pedaling in a small gear (90+ RPM), then stretching

CALORIES BURNED: About 47 calories per mile

COMMENTS

This is a good workout for moderately and highly fit cyclists who want to improve their climbing and their ability to recover quickly from hard efforts. Maintain the recommended HR during all phases, shifting as necessary.

WORKOUT 9

SPRINTS
TOTAL TIME: 55 minutes

9

WARM-UP: 15 minutes spinning at 90+ RPM, gradually increasing the gear

WORKOUT

Distance: 8-10 miles

Time: 30 minutes

Terrain: Flat to rolling road

Pace: Fast. Do 3-10 sprints—all-out efforts of 10-20 seconds with full recovery between sprints. Maintain a cadence of 90-110 RPM.

Effort: 90+% max HR during work phase

COOL-DOWN: 10 minutes easy pedaling in a small gear (90+ RPM), then stretching

CALORIES BURNED: About 55 calories per mile

COMMENTS

To build power, start your sprints from a near stop or at the bottom of a short hill; to build speed, sprint from a rolling start or on a slight descent. Recover fully between sprints.

10

INTERVALS
STATIONARY BIKE

TOTAL TIME: 50 minutes

WARM-UP: 15 minutes at 90+ RPM—5 minutes at zero resistance, 5 minutes at light resistance, 5 minutes at moderate resistance

WORKOUT

Time: 30 minutes

Resistance: Moderate to high during work intervals, light during rest. Ride hard for 15 seconds, then rest for 45 seconds. Perform this sequence 6 times with full recovery between each. Do 5 sets. Maintain a cadence of 90-100 RPM.

Effort: 90+% max HR during work phase

COOL-DOWN: 5 minutes easy pedaling at light resistance (90+ RPM), then stretching

CALORIES BURNED: About 13-15 calories per minute during high intensity phases

COMMENTS

This is a good workout for highly and moderately fit cyclists who want to improve their ability to cycle intensely. Done at high resistance, it can increase power; at moderate to light resistance, it can increase pedal cadence and speed.

	Summary Table Orange Zone Workouts			
Workout	**Description**	**Duration**	**Distance**	**Intensity**
1	Intervals on flat road	10 minutes	3.5 miles	75-90% max HR
2	Intervals on rolling hills	10 minutes	2.5 miles	75-90% max HR
3	Intervals on long hill	10 minutes	2 miles	75-90% max HR
4	Speedplay on flat to rolling hills	30 minutes	9-11 miles	90% max HR
5	Intervals at moderate to high intensity	30 minutes	—	75-90% max HR
6	Time trial on flat to rolling hills	30 minutes	10 miles	80-90% max HR
7	Time trial on moderately steep hill	30 minutes	5 miles	80-90% max HR
8	Climb on varied terrain with short, steep hills	30 minutes	7-9 miles	85-90% max HR
9	Hard sprints on flat to rolling road	30 minutes	8-10 miles	90+% max HR
10	Intervals at moderate to high intensity	30 minutes	—	90+% max HR

11

Red Zone

The Red zone, like a red light, should serve as a warning—stop and think about the state of your fitness before selecting one of these high-intensity, long-duration workouts, which will require you to work at 80 to 90 percent of your maximum heart rate for long periods of time. Perceived exertion on the RPE scale will be 7+, or very heavy.

The Red zone includes long intervals that serve as a good base for the shorter, more intense intervals in the second half of the Orange zone. These workouts, on flat, rolling, and hilly routes, will help you process oxygen more efficiently, enabling you to ride farther and faster with less perceived effort. Done on the flats, they will increase your average speed; on hills, they will augment your power and improve your climbing ability. They also can be done in sets, a type of workout recommended only for the highly fit. If you choose to do these workouts on a stationary bike, increase the resistance for the work phase, then decrease it for the rest phase. Recover completely between sets.

The Red zone also includes two race-pace efforts, a 25-mile time trial and a 90-minute "road race" to simulate the stress of competition—but don't think of them as for racers only. The power of a time trialist and the snap of a sprinter are useful for all cyclists, from casual riders to commuters.

The road race workout will require you to ride in a pace line—a group of cyclists who take turns "pulling" at the front and "drafting" in the leaders' slipstream. By doing this, they alternate hard work with rest and can actually travel a good deal faster with less effort than a solo cyclist. It takes practice; your local cycling club can show you the ropes.

The time trial effort, in which you race yourself and the clock, will help you increase your average speed over a preset course and give you some idea how you might fare in racing, either as an unlicensed racer or in U.S. Cycling Federation (USCF) or National Off-Road Bicycle Association (NORBA) competition. If you want to be a better climber, make your course a shorter, hilly one; if you want to ride farther and faster, select a flat route.

The Red zone workouts make excellent Wednesday, Saturday, or Sunday rides for moderately to highly fit cyclists.

WORKOUT 1

INTERVALS
TOTAL TIME: 1 hour 25 minutes

1

WARM-UP: 15 minutes spinning, gradually increasing the gear (90+ RPM)

WORKOUT

Distance: 19-21 miles

Time: 1 hour

Terrain: Flat road

Pace: Variable. Ride 2 minutes at 85-90% of your max HR, then rest for 6 minutes at 70-75% max HR. Perform this sequence 5 times. Then ride 20 minutes at 80% of your max HR. Maintain a cadence of 90-110 RPM.

Effort: 80-90% max HR

COOL-DOWN: 10 minutes easy pedaling in a small gear (90+ RPM), then stretching

CALORIES BURNED: About 50-60 calories per mile during intervals

COMMENTS

If you want to improve your speed, increase your cadence (to 100-110 RPM) rather than your gearing; if you need more power, upshift and maintain the 90 RPM cadence. Done in sets of 5 to 7 repetitions, with the less intense postinterval ride reduced to 6 to 8 minutes, it also makes a good workout for the highly fit.

WORKOUT 2

2

INTERVALS
TOTAL TIME: 1 hour 25 minutes

WARM-UP: 15 minutes spinning, gradually increasing the gear (90+ RPM)

WORKOUT

Distance: 15 miles

Time: 1 hour

Terrain: Rolling road

Pace: Variable. Ride 2 minutes at 85-90% of your max HR, then rest for 6 minutes at 70-75% max HR. Perform this sequence 6 times. Then ride 12 minutes at 80% of your max HR. Maintain a cadence of 90-110 RPM.

Effort: 80-90% max HR

COOL-DOWN: 10 minutes easy pedaling in a small gear (90+ RPM), then stretching

CALORIES BURNED: About 50-60 calories per mile during intervals

COMMENTS

If you want to improve your speed, increase your cadence; if you need more power, upshift. Done in sets with the less intense postinterval ride reduced to 6 to 8 minutes, this also makes a good workout for the highly fit.

WORKOUT 3

INTERVALS
TOTAL TIME: 1 hour 25 minutes

3

WARM-UP: 15 minutes spinning, gradually increasing the gear (90+ RPM)

WORKOUT

Distance: 15 miles

Time: 1 hour

Terrain: Long hill (moderate to steep)

Pace: Variable. Ride 3 minutes at 80-85% max HR, then rest for 9 minutes at 70-75% max HR. Perform this sequence 5 times. Maintain a cadence of 70-90 RPM.

Effort: 70-85% max HR

COOL-DOWN: 10 minutes easy pedaling in a small gear (90+ RPM), then stretching

CALORIES BURNED: About 50-60 calories per mile during work phase

COMMENTS

This is a good power-building workout. Remain seated as much as possible. When you must stand for a steep section, upshift to keep your workload steady, then downshift once you resume sitting.

WORKOUT 4

4

SPEEDPLAY
TOTAL TIME: 1 hour 55 minutes

WARM-UP: 15 minutes spinning, gradually increasing the gear (90+ RPM)

WORKOUT

Distance: 25 miles

Time: 1 hour 30 minutes

Terrain: Flat to rolling road

Pace: Fast. Ride in a pace line with a group, taking turns pulling at the front and drafting the other riders. Each rider should "attack" the group periodically, forcing the others to chase. Maintain a cadence of 90-110 RPM.

Effort: 90% max HR during work phases, 80-85% max HR at other times

COOL-DOWN: 10 minutes easy pedaling in a small gear (90+ RPM), then stretching.

CALORIES BURNED: About 50-60 calories per mile during intervals

COMMENTS

These high-intensity, race-pace efforts are much more fun than solo intervals, but achieve the same results. Attacking hills will force you to improve your power and climbing, whereas attacking flats or descents will force you to increase your cadence, acceleration, and overall speed.

WORKOUT 5

TIME TRIAL

TOTAL TIME: 1 hour 30 minutes

5

WARM-UP: 15 minutes at 90+ RPM. Begin with easy pedaling in a small gear, then add a few hard, big-gear efforts after 10 minutes.

WORKOUT

Distance: 25 miles

Time: About 1 hour

Terrain: Flat road

Pace: Fast. Time trial on a 12.5-mile, out-and-back course. Maintain a cadence of 90+ RPM.

Effort: 80-90% max HR

COOL-DOWN: 15 minutes easy pedaling in a small gear (90+ RPM), then stretching

CALORIES BURNED: About 38 calories per mile if cycling at 20 mph, 47 calories per mile if cycling at 25 mph, or 60 calories per mile if cycling at 30 mph

COMMENTS

Select a 12.5-mile course with minimal traffic. Warm up for 15 minutes by riding in a small gear, then time yourself over the distance, turning around at the 12.5-mile point and returning to the start. Select a gear that lets you pedal smoothly at the specified HR for the entire distance. Begin by riding at 80% of your max HR, then increase the intensity with successive workouts until you reach the maximum of 90%. You should see your time decrease as the weeks fly by. (Note that once a week is plenty for this type of strenuous effort.) This workout will give you an idea of what racing is like. Riding 25 miles in an hour or less is an indicator that you could be competitive in USCF racing, where the official championship time trial distance is 40 kilometers—about 25 miles.

WORKOUT 6

TIME TRIAL
STATIONARY BIKE

TOTAL TIME: 1 hour 30 minutes

WARM-UP: 15 minutes spinning, gradually increasing resistance

WORKOUT

Time: About 1 hour
Resistance: High
Effort: 80-85% max HR

COOL-DOWN: 15 minutes easy pedaling at low resistance (90+ RPM), then stretching

CALORIES BURNED: About 13-15 calories per minute

COMMENTS

Keep the intensity high, occasionally accelerating for about 20-30 seconds. Every 10-15 minutes ride out of the saddle in a slightly higher resistance for about 90 seconds.

Summary Table Red Zone Workouts				
Workout	**Description**	**Duration**	**Distance**	**Intensity**
1	Intervals on flat road	1 hour	19-21 miles	80-90% max HR
2	Intervals on rolling road	1 hour	15 miles	80-90% max HR
3	Intervals on long hill	1 hour	15 miles	70-85% max HR
4	Speedplay on flat to rolling road	1 hour 30 minutes	25 miles	80-90% max HR
5	Time trial on flat road	1 hour	25 miles	80-90% max HR
6	Time trial at high intensity	1 hour	—	80-85% max HR

PART III

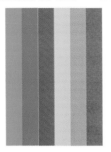

TRAINING BY THE WORKOUT ZONES

Now that you've been introduced to the workouts, the chapters in this part will help you learn how to use them in a training program.

Think of the color-coded workouts in this book as a smorgasbord—instead of sticking with a single exercise entree, you can choose from throughout the various zones a variety of workouts suited to your aerobic appetite.

Chapter 12 provides some guidelines for you to use as you set up your cycling program. Chapter 13 provides sample programs. You can use them as they are or modify them to meet your goals and needs. Chapter 14 discusses the benefits of cross-training and suggests several activities for your off-the-bike days. Chapter 15 provides a training log to help you record your workouts—and your progress.

The cycling efficiency test you took in chapter 3 will help you decide where to begin. The sample programs are based on three levels of interest and ability:

- **Beginning/easy:** These programs pull workouts from primarily the low-intensity zones. They are geared toward those who are just beginning to ride or who are interested in cycling for exercise and aerobic benefit. If the cycling efficiency test indicated your fitness level is currently below average, consider starting with these beginning programs. If they are too difficult, then begin with the low-intensity short-duration spins of the Green zone to raise your fitness level.
- **Frequent/moderate:** These programs pull workouts from the low- and medium-intensity zones. They are geared toward those interested in cycling a little harder and more frequently than in the previous level. If the test indicates you're moderately fit, you're probably ready to try these programs.
- **Competitive/intense:** These programs pull workouts from all levels, concentrating efforts in the medium- and high-intensity zones. They are designed for those who like to ride hard, fast, and often. If you are an experienced cyclist, or if the efficiency test indicated that you are highly fit, you may relish the challenge posed by these programs.

Whether you use the samples in chapter 13 or create your own program, remember that you don't have to use the workouts in a progressive manner unless you want to. Your enjoyment will come from using the variety of the workouts in a way that best fits your goals and your abilities. Experiment to see what's best for you.

12

Setting Up Your Program

Designing a workout program involves walking a fine line between exercise and rest. You want to work hard enough to challenge your cardiopulmonary system, but not so hard that you risk illness or injury from overtraining. Resist the temptation to exercise vigorously every day—it will hinder your development, not accelerate it. Make your weekly schedule a healthy blend of hard rides, easy spins, and days off.

Start Hard, Finish Easy

In designing your weekly schedule, begin with your most intense workout and move to less taxing rides. You won't have the snap to do a tough Red zone workout if you did some taxing Orange zone intervals the day before. The sample schedules in chapter 13 show how to mix hard and easy workouts.

Take a Break

Regardless of your fitness level, consider taking 1 day completely off the bike. Racers who compete on Sunday generally choose Monday as their rest day; you may want to do the same if you choose to do a long, intense Red zone ride on Sunday.

Add at least one "active rest" day during the week. This means riding at a low intensity to help tired muscles recover from a previous day's hard efforts. The Green and Blue zones include suitable active rest rides for the moderately and highly fit; you might choose to do one of them on Friday if you plan a hard Orange zone ride on Saturday.

Elements of a Training Program

Different training methods yield different results. If you train by doing only long, steady miles on the flats, that's all you're going to be able to ride—abrupt changes in pace or elevation may have you gasping for air like a first-timer. If your training consists of short, intense rides, you may be able to hammer for a while, but 20 miles into a 50-mile ride, you may be ready to keel over.

A successful training program consists of a variety of workouts. This not only trains your body for different efforts, it keeps your mind interested in the sport. If you use the same old routine, you won't keep riding.

We've already introduced several different types of rides in chapters 6 to 11. Here we'll discuss in more detail the benefits of each type of ride to help you determine how to incorporate them into your cycling program.

Long, Steady Distance

Low-intensity rides provide you with an aerobic base on which you construct all other elements of your exercise program. Many top cyclists ride little else for the first 2 months of the season as they rebuild from time spent off the bike. These low-intensity rides burn fat and strengthen your heart and lungs, allowing them to deliver more oxygen to your muscles. They also strengthen muscles new to cycling (or just back from a vacation).

Intervals

High-intensity intervals come in two varieties—aerobic and anaerobic. Both enable you to work at a higher-than-normal intensity for brief periods by alternating work phases, or intervals, with rest phases. But each uses a different fuel. Aerobic intervals tend to be longer efforts; they remain within the aerobic range, both in the work and rest phase, and use oxygen to burn fatty acids. Anaerobic intervals are short, hard efforts that cross your anaerobic threshold, after which your body can't deliver oxygen fast enough for muscles to burn fat. Muscles then begin to feed on anaerobic glycogen and generate lactic acid (along with a corresponding amount of pain).

Aerobic intervals provide a shortcut toward stronger heart, lungs, and legs. If you work hard for short periods on a regular basis, you soon will be able to work hard for longer periods. Anaerobic intervals help boost

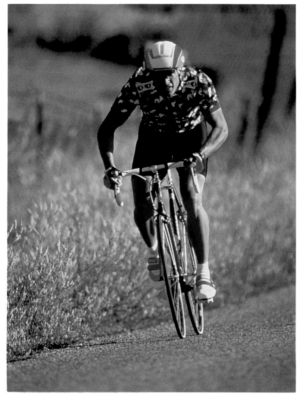

John Kelly/Courtesy Pearl Izumi

Interval training can increase power and speed.

your anaerobic threshold, meaning that you can ride longer and harder without going into oxygen debt and reaching exhaustion (known to cyclists as "blowing up").

Why do intervals? Because cycling rarely demands a single level of effort. Climbing hills demands power; getting home before a heavy snowfall requires speed. Regular interval training can give you power and speed.

Sprints

Sprints are speed, pure and simple. Done at nearly 100% of your maximum heart rate, they can help you win a race or get through a crowded intersection before the light turns red. Sprints increase the efficiency of your fast-twitch muscle fibers and improve your body's ability to use the high-energy adenosine triphosphate stored in its tissues. The results are increased strength and power and faster reaction time. Adding a weekly sprint session to your program can give you the leg speed you'll need to catch the postman with that overdue bill or to get away from a loose and toothy dog. Also, they're fun.

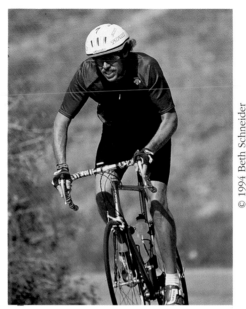

Listen to your body.

Time Trials

Time trials are races against yourself and the clock. Choose a course with minimal traffic and ride it weekly or monthly, under similar weather conditions when possible, and chart your times. Cycling clubs often conduct regular series of time trials, and it's fun to check your times against those of your friends. It's good training in that trying to better your time from the previous week will have you riding a little harder over your course. Also, timing yourself over the same course on a regular basis can tell you how well your exercise program is proceeding.

Modifying Your Schedule

As your fitness improves, you may want to expand the duration and intensity of your workouts. If you've been taking a day off each Friday, but the down time leaves you sluggish for Saturday's workout, you may decide to do an easy Green zone spin on Friday as a recovery ride. Conversely, if you feel fatigued after a hard Yellow zone workout on Wednesday and face a hard Red zone workout on Thursday, you might instead take a day off, or substitute a less intense Blue zone spin.

The key? Listen to your body. It's the best judge of how to proceed. And periodically retake the cycling efficiency test you used to determine your fitness, being sure to ride the same bicycle on the same course under comparable environmental conditions. It will help you chart your progress and make any necessary adjustments in your training program.

The Yearly Program

Cycling, like any other sport, has a season and an off-season. And even if you live in a climate that permits cycling year-round, you should have an off-season, too. The phrase "too much of a good thing" can apply to riding a bike. If you're burned out on biking, you won't ride, and all the training programs in the world won't do you a bit of good.

The Preseason: January-February

Start your year gradually, with low-intensity spinning to develop aerobic conditioning, strength, and technique throughout January and February. If you live in snow country, you may not be able to ride outdoors as much as you like. But you can always break out the stationary bike or substitute ice skating, cross-country skiing, or running until the weather clears. If you choose the stationary bike, be sure to set up a fan to keep cool, and have plenty of water handy.

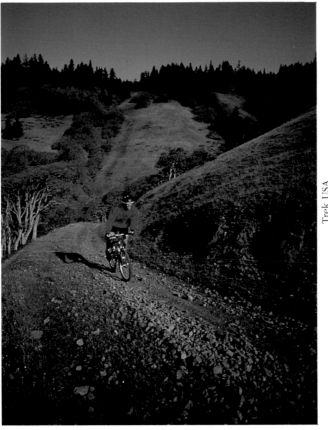

Trek USA

Mixing up your workouts will keep your riding interesting.

The Season: March-October

Design a schedule of increments of 6 to 8 weeks with gradual increases in duration and intensity. At the end of each period, take a few days off from cycling to recuperate before resuming your training at an intensity and duration slightly below that which ended the previous period.

Begin your season by logging a few weeks of spinning on the flats to rebuild your aerobic base, then head for the hills to give yourself a little more intensity. Mix up your workouts with flat rides, hilly rides, and long and short intervals to build endurance and power; also try occasional self-testing time trials like the cycling efficiency test described in chapter 3. You'll build strength gradually and safely without the boredom that comes from doing the same thing regularly.

Set a goal, such as riding the Red zone time trial 15 seconds faster than you did last month, or completing a 50-mile ride organized by your local cycling club. You can design a program of gradually increasing duration and intensity that will help you peak in time for your event. But if you get sick or have an injury, don't panic—recover adequately, then resume training gradually. Trying to ride through an injury or illness can exacerbate the problem and actually do more damage than not training at all. Listen to your body.

The Off-Season: November-December

Take a long break—as much as a month if you like—then continue to ride a few times each week at reduced intensity while cross-training with such sports as running, in-line or ice skating, cross-country skiing, snow-shoeing, or weightlifting (see chapter 14). Running, diagonal-stride skiing, and snowshoeing can serve as substitutes for long endurance rides; ice or in-line skating and the skating method of cross-country skiing, which are more closely related to cycling, can be used to create interval and speed workouts similar to those done on the bike. These activities will complement and enhance your cycling for the coming year while giving you a much-needed rest from the past year's efforts.

13

Sample Cycling Programs

The following are examples of how to set up a training program based upon your beginning level of fitness. We have also devised programs within each fitness level for those cyclists wanting to work primarily on endurance and another set of workouts for those who want to add speed or more intensity to their programs. You may also want to combine programs; for example, follow an endurance program for 3 weeks and then throw in a week of speedwork.

Beginning/Easy Cycling Programs

As a beginning cyclist, you work out for the enjoyment and/or the aerobic benefits. But the endless laps around a city park are getting boring. The beginning/easy schedules that follow will add some variety to your cycling routine. They offer four workouts per week from primarily the low-intensity zones.

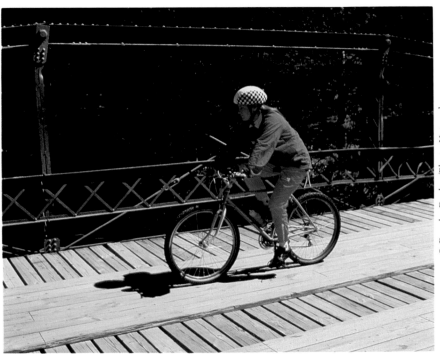

© Brooks Dodge/Photo Network

A beginning cyclist, enjoying the benefits of the sport.

Building Endurance

This program is for the cyclist who wants to build endurance so that he or she can ride comfortably at a steady pace for 1 hour or more. The cyclist may want to be able to ride with the local bike club on weekends or occasionally take a 20- to 25-mile ride on the weekends after several months of riding and conditioning.

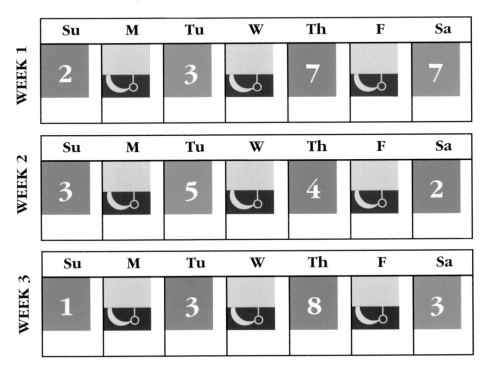

	Su	M	Tu	W	Th	F	Sa
WEEK 1	2		3		7		7
WEEK 2	3		5		4		2
WEEK 3	1		3		8		3

Building Speed

You may occasionally want to ride faster for increased anaerobic capacity, to build speed and strength, or because you want to work a little harder. The following sample demonstrates a speed-building program.

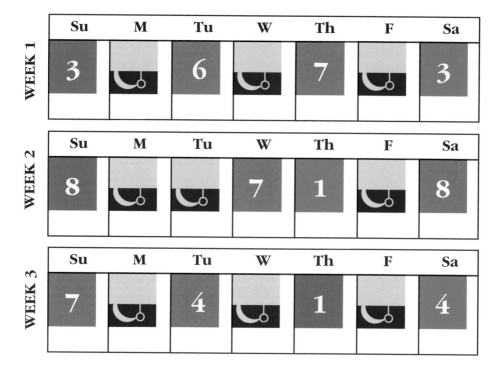

Frequent/Moderate Cycling Programs

As a frequent cyclist, you take the next step beyond the beginning level. You may have ambitions of completing a long weekend tour (50 miles or more) in 1 day. The frequent/moderate schedules that follow offer 5 workouts per week, mixing workouts from primarily the low- and medium-intensity zones.

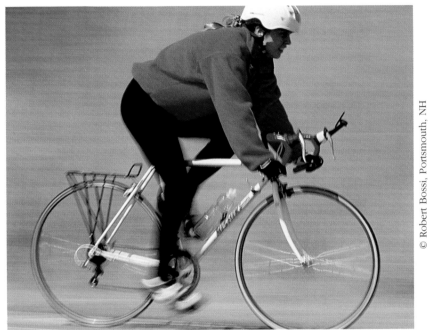

© Robert Bossi, Portsmouth, NH

A frequent cyclist, testing her limits.

Building Endurance

This program is based on building endurance with moderate intensity. You will be riding longer distances and putting in more time on the bicycle. You will be resting only 2 days a week.

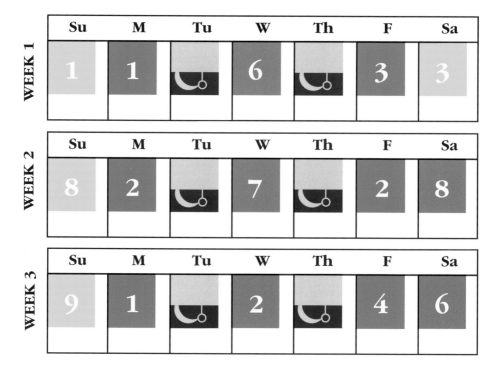

Building Speed

You ride for fitness and for fun, too—and you'd like to get a little faster, a little stronger. Here's how you might put together a 3-week schedule that gradually increases in intensity by blending workouts from a variety of zones with 2 days of off-the-bike rest.

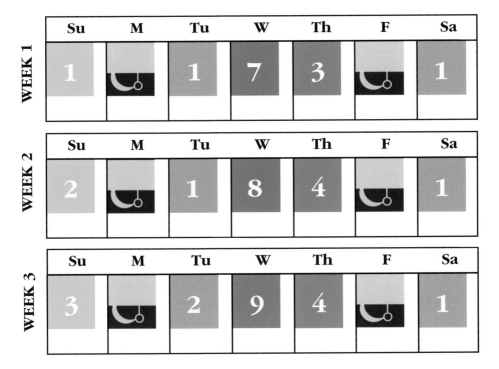

Variation. In week 2, consider adding an additional set to your intervals (Orange Workout 1). In week 3, add 1 or 2 additional sets, depending on how you feel.

Competitive/Intense Cycling Programs

As a competitive cyclist, you like to ride hard, fast, and often. The term *competitive* really means you're competing with yourself and your previous cycling performances. But you may be thinking about entering your first citizen's race or riding your first century ride (100 miles). The competitive/intense schedules offer 5 to 6 workouts per week and use workouts from all zones.

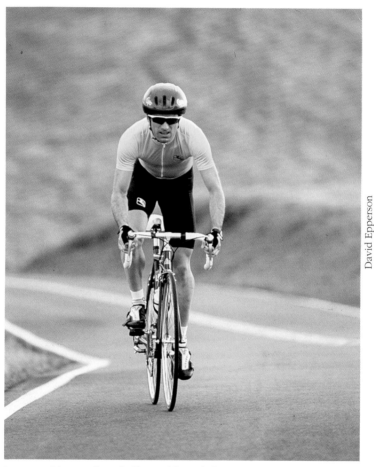

David Epperson

A competitive cyclist, challenged by a hill.

Building Endurance

This schedule focuses on longer distance rides, but it also includes rides of higher intensities. Note that you're often asked to lengthen your rides by repeating workouts. When a workout is to be repeated, the workout number will be followed by the number of repetitions, for example, (×2).

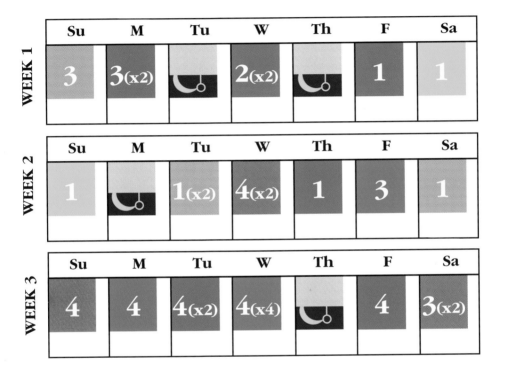

Building Speed

This schedule mixes workouts from all six zones. It gradually increases in intensity toward a time trial, then eases off a little to give you some recovery before you resume riding.

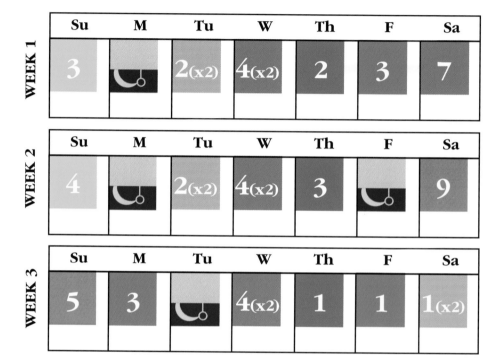

Variation.   Ride 6 repetitions during your interval and climbing workouts (Orange Workout 2 and Purple Workout 4) in week 1. In week 2, increase the number of repetitions to 7. In week 3, return to 5 repetitions per workout.

14

Cross-Training

Serious cyclists ride in all kinds of conditions, from driving rain to freezing snow—but you don't have to. When the weather or your motivation turns sour, leave the bike in the garage and try something a little bit different.

You can choose among a variety of activities to complement your cycling training, whether you want to augment the bike work or simply need a change of pace. Running, cross-country skiing, and weight training are the most common alternatives, but in-line skating and snowshoeing are becoming almost as popular. Each of these fitness activities works many of the same muscle groups used in cycling, but in a different way. Thus, cross-training prevents road-weary cyclists from becoming stale while maintaining, and even enhancing, their fitness levels and muscular strength. This translates to improved cycling when you do feel like riding. Cross-training also works muscle groups that cycling ignores, which will help you create a more well-rounded physique.

A word of caution: Start any new exercise gradually. You may feel fit, and indeed you may be—for cycling. But different exercises use different muscle groups, and if you overdo it, you'll pay afterward with soreness or even injury.

Running

Long-distance running is a great training alternative, and a quick way to build leg and lung power. Best of all, unlike cycling, it's low-tech; all you need is a good pair of shoes.

A long run can provide a terrific aerobic workout, especially when combined with riding, either outdoors on the road or indoors on a stationary bike. A short run can keep your fitness from ebbing if for one reason or another—work, travel, or weather—you're unable to ride. Just a half-hour run can give you a workout equivalent to 2 hours on the bike.

Inclement weather is less of a roadblock to running than riding, since you're out for less time and generating a lot of heat. Also, you don't have to worry about navigating your bike over slick pavement or through puddles. Trails, gravel running paths, or dirt roads are better than concrete or asphalt surfaces. Running uphill is best of all, but remember to slow to a jog or even a walk on the descents. Otherwise, you'll wake up the next morning with some awfully sore leg muscles (hamstrings and gastrocnemius) that your cycling training doesn't tax.

If your body is accustomed to the stress of running, you can add some workouts that will contribute to developing your cardiovascular system and the power muscles of cycling, the quadriceps. Your high school football stadium can provide an excellent interval workout—run up the stairs to the top, then walk or jog back down to recover. Repeat until your speed noticeably slows. Your favorite mountain-bike trail can be a great running course—push the pace on the uphills, then walk or jog the descents.

When running on the flats or rolling trails, start with a brisk walk to warm up (about 10 minutes), then move into a jogging pace. Continue at an easy pace for 20 minutes, alternating running and walking, then cool down by walking for 5 to 10 minutes. Stretch afterward. Continue with the 20-minute duration until you can run for the entire period; then, next time out, try a slightly faster pace and a 25-minute run. Increase your duration by 5 minutes per workout over the next several weeks until you can run for an hour. Give yourself at least 1 day in between runs to recover—running is harder on the tissues than cycling.

Cross-Country Skiing

This is a popular mode of exercise with pro cyclists and top amateurs. The skating technique exercises the same lower-body muscle groups used in cycling, maintains and extends aerobic power, and adds an upper-body workout as you use the ski poles to augment the efforts being made by your legs.

When done for 30 minutes or more, skiing is a terrific aerobic workout. You'll get your heart rate up quickly because you are using both your arms and your legs. If you've skied downhill before, you're halfway there; if you've never been on skis, or never tried the skating method of cross-country skiing, plan on taking a lesson or two from a teacher certified by the Professional Ski Instructors of America.

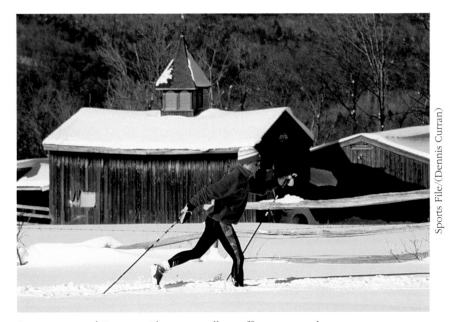

Cross-country skiing provides an excellent off-season workout.

You can rent equipment at most Nordic skiing areas, and unless you're certain cross-country skiing is going to be one of your cross-training activities, renting is the best option—equipping yourself with everything you'll need, from skis to boots to bindings to poles, will cost you a minimum of $300. As with running, start slowly, adding intensity and endurance as you gain proficiency. As with cycling, you can "ski" indoors—devices such as the Nordic Track® can give you an excellent workout, using both the upper and lower body, without the hazards of the real thing.

Weight Training

A weight program can be an excellent off-season way to develop the leg power you need as a cyclist. It can also tone some of the areas of the body that cycling ignores and help prevent injury.

Here, as with other cross-training exercises, the key is to start small. Gradual progression from low percentages of your maximum 1 rep lifts is the best method. Overdoing a weight program will leave you too sore to do anything else for days.

Consult a certified strength and conditioning specialist at your local YMCA or health club. And be sure to get a good aerobic warm-up before lifting—jog, pedal a stationary bike, anything to warm up the muscles and break a light sweat. Stretch afterward.

Begin with circuit training twice a week on a multigym or circuit setup. You want to quickly go through a series of exercises for the lower body, torso, and upper body. Squats build the quads while working the glutes and lower back; leg curls help strengthen the hamstrings, which cycling neglects; and heel raises build the major muscles of the calf. Each exercise should take 20 to 40 seconds and should be followed by recovery intervals of 10 seconds to a minute as you move to the next workout. Begin with light weights and 10 to 15 repetitions for each exercise, and alternately work different body parts—for example, a bench press for the upper body, followed by abdominal crunches and squats for the legs. Repeat the complete circuit at least once; after a month of steady lifting, think about adding a third circuit.

If you want to build power, add progressive sets. Do your first set with a weight you can handle comfortably for 10 or more reps, rest 30 seconds to a minute, than do a second set with a weight that will fatigue you in 6 to 10 reps. After a month of progressive sets, increase the weight or add a third set.

In-Line Skating

The fastest-growing sport in the nation, in-line skating uses many of the same muscle groups employed in cycling. This is not just a fad, but a legitimate fitness activity that stresses the lower-body muscles. You can start by renting equipment at your local skate shop; if you like in-line skating enough to buy your own skates, expect to pay $100 or more for a serviceable pair.

Take a lesson or two from an International In-Line Skating Association–certified instructor near you. Many skate shops employ certified instructors, and they can give you a few pointers on the most difficult part of skating—stopping. The 4-wheeled skates you rolled around on as a kid had a brake on each toe, but today's in-line versions have only one, on the right heel, and it takes some getting used to.

As in cycling, safety gear is a must. Wear the same helmet you use on your bike, then add wrist guards ($15 and up), knee pads ($20 and up), and elbow pads ($15 and up). If you're going to cut corners on cost, at least get the wrist guards. The most common skating injury, besides skinned knees and elbows, is a broken wrist.

Begin on a flat, traffic-free pavement. Church parking lots during the week and shopping mall parking lots after hours are great. Practice stopping first, then add corners and gradual hills (you can slalom the

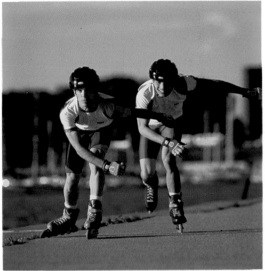

© 1994 Mark D. Maziarz

Try in-line skating for a change of pace.

descents to keep your speed manageable). Once you become proficient at descending, cornering, and stopping, you can move to the streets or your neighborhood park.

As with running, push the pace on hills and recover on the descents—you'll build leg power that will serve you well once you return to the bike. Add a set of poles with carbide tips for pounding the pavement on uphills and you can get the same upper-body workout as a cross-country skier.

Snowshoeing

If you think of snowshoes as heavy, bulky affairs best suited to trudging across Alaska, think again. Today's snowshoes use aluminum and Hypalon, not leather and wood. In fact, they're not that much bigger than running shoes, which is what you wear underneath the laces-and-Velcro bindings of today's lightweight snowshoes. And yes, you can run with these high-tech snowshoes, but it's not necessary. Simply "post-holing" through the drifts, especially if you head uphill, is enough to send your heart rate through the roof.

Many top amateur cyclists are using snowshoeing for their endurance workouts during the winter months. It's a great cardiovascular workout, but easier on the legs than running. Don't let that fool you, though; pulling your snowshoe back up through the snow will use more calf muscle than bike riding. And if you overdo a snowshoe workout, you'll feel it in the calves the next day. As with skates, you can rent before you buy. If you decide to purchase your own pair of snowshoes, expect to pay $150 or more.

15

Charting Your Progress

About 50% of all those who begin an exercise program drop out within 6 months. In addition, only about 20% of the population exercises regularly enough to be considered fit by government statistics. How do we stop from becoming a bad statistic?

While we all have good intentions, these have little to do with people sticking with an exercise program. Success in a cycling fitness program depends on attitude, personality, and logistics. You should enjoy exercising and make it convenient enough to stick with it. You also should believe that exercise will make a positive difference in your life.

It helps to have the support of your friends, spouse, and family. Make sure your close friends and family support your efforts and are not inconvenienced by your cycling. If you decide to cycle after work, this may change the routine of your whole family. You need to anticipate this in advance and work something out for dinner or child care.

Lack of time is the most frequent excuse for not riding your bike. How does a parent with a full-time job find time to exercise? Logistics are the barrier for most of us.

We advise you to find a convenient time and location for cycling, and lock it into your schedule three or four times a week. Make exercise as important as having lunch with your boss. Once again, enlisting friends who will count on you to ride with them or joining a cycling club may improve your motivation. If weather is a problem, we have given you many suggestions for indoor cycling on a stationary bicycle or wind-load simulator.

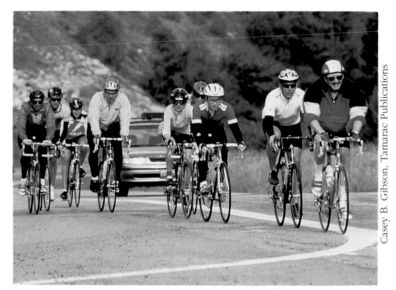

Group rides offer a sense of community and friendly competition.

Casey B. Gibson, Tamarac Publications

Boredom is another reason people become exercise casualties. Variation is the key. Follow the suggestions we've provided and vary your training among the color-coded zones. Have several routes you can use for training. Ride with a friend and discuss the latest developments in the news. When riding indoors watch television, listen to music, or read a magazine. Go out for a leisurely ride and don't worry about heart rate or distance traveled.

Try something different by following our suggestions in chapter 14. Try in-line skating, go swimming, climb a mountain, or try Alpine skiing. The possibilities are limited only by your imagination.

Develop Sound Goals

It will be helpful for you to set some goals as you begin a cycling program. Good goals can help motivate you to stick with your exercise program and challenge you to push yourself a little harder. And it's a great feeling to set a goal and watch yourself achieve it!

As you set your goals, follow these guidelines:

- Make your goals challenging, but realistic. Rather than setting a goal of riding a century ride (100-mile tour) it may be a more appropriate goal to ride 25 miles in 1 day at the end of 4 months.

- Set specific, not general, goals. Don't set a goal that says "to improve my cycling performance." Instead, for example, aim to increase your cycling speed over a known course after so many weeks of training.
- Set goals that you can reach within a time period that is short enough to keep you motivated. For example, if your goal is to lose 30 pounds while cycling this year, set a goal to lose 3 pounds this month.

Take a few minutes to think about your personal goals. After you have identified some, write them down. Then, as you continue in your exercise program, your list will help remind you of how much you have achieved. You may have to adjust your goals after you complete your cycling efficiency test.

Check Your Progress

Keeping track of your progress in your cycling fitness program is like checking the highway signs on a cross-country cycling trip—it helps you know exactly where you are.

Keeping records only takes a few seconds every day, but it's very important for your total fitness program. It takes the guesswork out of trying to remember what you did and how you felt each time you rode outdoors or indoors. Every time you record your progress, you show yourself how far you've come. You'll also want to refer back periodically to the goals you've set to determine when you reach them. If you have met a goal, set a new one. It will be easier to stay with your cycling exercise program when you can see the progress you've made.

We hope you can see how easy it will be for you to use this book and to participate in a cycling fitness program. We've done all the planning for you so that you can put all your energy into riding your bicycle.

Measure Your Progress

Log your workouts and accomplishments as you progress toward your goals. If you are trying to lose weight, get on a scale once a week and post your results on the refrigerator. Take photos of yourself every few months in your cycling clothes and put them with your training diary to document the improvements in your body composition.

Keeping a log of your training and other fitness accomplishments can be very helpful. Some people find that recording the date, the miles ridden, how long the ride took, and how they feel is all they need to keep informed and motivated. But as you become more experienced, we believe you'll want to keep more details.

We recommend a training log similar to the one shown on p.157. You could either photocopy this page or adopt a similar one. Keep your training goals with your training log. With a log, you'll be able to chart your progress. You'll notice changes: Your weight will go down. Your resting pulse will decrease. And you will need harder workouts to get your heart rate into your target heart rate zone.

Although it may take a few minutes to fill out the log before or after your workout, it's worth it. You'll be able to look back at where you were 1 or 2 years ago, and realize how far you've come, and how fit you are.

Reward Yourself

Finally, many people forget to stop and give themselves a well-deserved pat on the back for a job well done. If you have started exercising and complete a month, if you win your first race, or set a personal best time in a local time trial, buy yourself a present. Get something you have been wanting a long time. After 4 months, if you keep with your program, take your spouse or a friend out to dinner. Simple rewards remind you that you are the one in charge and that your hard work is improving your quality of life.

Most of all, remember that your cycling program can very easily lead to a more active and healthy lifestyle. It involves simple planning and a desire to exercise that makes cycling a natural, fun part of our lives.

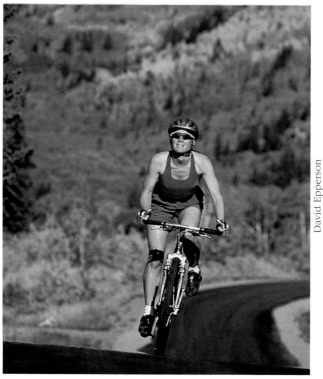

David Epperson

Training is its own reward.

Date	Pulse Weight		Workout zone and #	Distance	Time	Comments
Su						
M						
Tu						
W						
Th						
F						
Sa						

Summary _____

_____

_____

_____

Index

A

Achilles tendon stretching exercise, 42
Adductor stretching exercise, 43
Aerobic exercise. *See also* Aerobic interval
    workouts; Aerobics, compared to
    cycling
  cross-training for, 148, 149
  cycling in general as, 5, 9
  definition of, 132
  specific zone workouts for, 65, 79
Aerobic interval workouts
  basic guidelines, 93
  benefits of, 132
  yellow zone outdoor, 94-97, 99-102
Aerobics, compared to cycling, 8, 9
Age factors, 4, 24
Anaerobic threshold training. *See also*
    Interval workouts
  benefits of, 132-133
  definition of, 105, 132
Arm warmers, 19

B

Back, effects of uphill cycling on, 79
Back stretching exercise, 46
Beginning cycling programs, 130, 138-140
Benefits of cycling, 3, 4, 5-9, 132-134, 156
Bicycles
  adjustment of, 31-35
  selection/purchasing guidelines, 11-15
Blue zone workouts
  basic guidelines, 65-66
  specific intructions, 67-76
  summary table, 77
Body composition, 6
Body position. *See* Position for cycling
Body weight and fitness, 25
Borg, Gunnar, 51. *See also* RPE (Rating of
    Perceived Exertion)
Buttocks stretching exercise, 45

C

Cadence, pedaling. See Pedaling technique

Caloric output, 6
Cardiorespiratory fitness
  aerobic interval workouts for, 93, 94-97,
    99-102, 132
  general benefits of cycling for, 3, 5-6
Cardiovascular fitness, assessment of, 24
Charting progress, 155-156, 157
Climbing (uphill cycling)
  basic guidelines, 65-66, 79-80, 93, 120
  loops for workouts for, 65, 80
  steady climb workouts, 65-66, 72-75, 81
  variable intensity climb workouts, 82-84,
    96-97, 114
Clothing, 16-17, 18-19
Color-coding of workouts, explained, 49
Competitive cycling. *See also* Competitive/
    intense cycling programs; Time trial
    workouts
  aerobic interval workouts for, 93, 94-97,
    99-102, 132
  health benefits of, 4
  orange zone workouts for, 106, 110, 115
  purple zone workouts as warm-ups for,
    79
  red zone workouts for, 119-120, 124
  road race workouts for, 119-120, 124
  speedplay workouts for, 110, 119-120,
    124
  sprint workouts for, 106, 115, 133
Competitive/intense cycling programs, 130,
    144-146
Computer, handlebar, 18
Cooling down
  basic guidelines, 41
  from interval workouts, 105
  stretching exercises for, 41-47
Cooper, Kenneth, 9
Costs
  of cross-training equipment, 149, 150,
    151
  of cycling equipment, 14-15, 17, 18, 19,
    20-21

Cross-country skiing, 148-149
Cross-training
guidelines for specific types of, 147-151
motivational benefits of, 154
yearly scheduling of, 135, 136
Cycling efficiency test
basic guidelines, 27-29
checking progress with, 29, 134, 136
Cyclists, statistics on, 4, 5

D

Dehydration, prevention of, 22, 66
Dropping out, 153
Duathlons, 4

E

Efficiency test, 27-29
Endurance, workouts for building
aerobic intervals, 93, 94-97, 99-102, 132
blue zone outdoor, 67-70, 72-75
blue zone stationary, 71, 76
sample schedules, 139, 142, 145
steady climbs, 72-75
variable intensity, 67-71, 76
yellow zone outdoor, 94-97, 99-102
Equipment
bicycles, 11-15
clothing, 16-17, 18-19
costs of cycling equipment, 14-15, 17, 18, 19, 20-21
for cross-training, 147, 149, 150, 151
eyewear, 19
heart rate monitor, 19
helmets, 16
miscellaneous accessories, 18
shoes, 17
stationary bicycles, 15
wind trainers, 15
Exercise bicycles. See Stationary cycling
Eyewear, 19

F

Fitness checks
checking progress with, 29, 134
cycling efficiency test, 27-29, 134
maximal stress tests, 50-51
in program planning, 23, 27, 50-52
questionnaire, 23-27
Flat tires, equipment for fixing, 18
Flexibility, benefits of cycling for, 6
Flexibility exercises. See Stretching exercises
Foot position, bicycle adjustment for, 32

Frequent/moderate cycling programs, 130, 141-143

G

Gearing technique
for aerobic interval workouts, 93
basic guidelines, 36, 37
for blue zone workouts, 65, 66
for climbing (uphill cycling), 66, 80
during cool-down, 41
for green zone workouts, 53
for injury prevention, 106
for interval workouts, 105, 106
for sprints, 106
for time trials, 106
for variable intensity workouts, 80
Gloves, 16-17
Goal setting, 154-155
Green zone workouts
basic guidelines, 53
specific instructions, 54-63
summary table, 64
as warm-ups, 106

H

Hamstring stretching exercise, 43
Handlebar adjustment, 33-34
Handlebar computer, 18
Health history, 23-27
Heart rate
for blue zone workouts, 52, 65, 66, 77
for cool-downs, 41
equipment for monitoring, 19
in fitness assessment, 25
for green zone workouts, 52, 53, 64
for interval workouts, 105, 106
maximum heart rate, 50-51
for orange zone workouts, 52, 105, 106, 117
for purple zone workouts, 52, 79, 80, 91
for recovery, 106
for red zone workouts, 52, 119, 127
and selection of workout zones, 49, 51, 52
target heart rate, 51
techniques for measuring, 50
for variable intensity workouts, 80
for warm-ups, 40
for yellow zone workouts, 52, 93, 104
Helmets, 16
Hills, cycling on. See Climbing (uphill cycling)
Hip stretching exercises, 45

Hybrid style bicycles
    adjustment of, 34
    selection of, 13-14
Hydration, 22, 66

I

Illnesses, in fitness assessment, 24
Indoor cycling. See Stationary cycling
Injuries
    and cross-training, 147
    cycling technique for preventing, 36, 106
    exercise for preventing, 40, 41, 42, 149
    in fitness assessment, 24
    muscle strain/soreness, 42, 148
    saddle sores, 16
    scheduling training for recovery from,
        136
In-line skating, 150-151
Intense cycling programs, 130, 144-146
Intensity of training
    of blue zone workouts, 52, 65, 66, 77
    color-coding for, explained, 49
    of green zone workouts, 52, 53, 64
    of orange zone workouts, 52, 105, 117
    and pedaling/gearing technique, 36
    of purple zone workouts, 52, 79, 91
    of red zone workouts, 52, 119, 127
    and selection of workout zones, 49, 51,
        52
    techniques for measuring, 50-51
    of warm-ups, 40
    of workout zones, overview, 49, 50, 51,
        52
    of yellow zone workouts, 52, 93, 104
Interval workouts. See also Aerobic interval
        workouts
    basic guidelines, 105-106
    benefits of, 132-133
    orange zone outdoor, 107-109
    orange zone stationary, 111, 116
    red zone outdoor, 121-123

J

Jackets, 18
Jerseys, 18

K

Knees, stresses on, 36, 79

L

Laws on bicycling, 21-22
Leg position, bicycle adjustment for, 25
Leg warmers, 19
Locations for cycling, 21, 80
Log, of training progress, 155-156, 157

Loop locations for cycling, 65, 80
Lower back, effects of uphill cycling on, 79
Lower back stretching exercise, 46

M

Maximal stress tests, 50-51
Maximum heart rate, determination of, 50-
        51. See also Heart rate
Moderate cycling programs, 130, 141-143
Motivation, 153-154, 156. See also Benefits
        of cycling
Mountain bicycles
    adjustment of, 34
    selection of, 12-13
Muscle strain/soreness
    from running, 148
    stretching exercises for preventing, 42
Muscular fitness
    aerobic interval workouts for, 93, 94-97,
        99-102, 132
    benefits of cycling for, 3, 7, 8
    and pedaling/gearing technique, 36
    purple zone workouts for, 79
    steady ride workouts for, 132
    weight training for, 149-150

N

National Off-Road Bicycle Association
        (NORBA), 120
Neck stretching exercises, 46, 47

O

Off-season scheduling, 136
Orange zone workouts
    basic guidelines, 105-106
    specific instructions, 107-116
    summary table, 117

P

Pace line, 119-120
Pedaling technique
    for aerobic interval workouts, 93
    basic guidelines, 36, 37
    for blue zone workouts, 65
    for climbing (uphill cycling), 79, 80
    during cool-down, 41
    for green zone workouts, 53
    for interval workouts, 105, 106
    for stationary cycling, 79, 106
    for variable intensity workouts, 80
Perceived Exertion, Rating of (RPE). See
        RPE (Rating of Perceived Exertion)
Position for cycling
    benefits/importance of proper position,
        31, 37
    bicycle adjustment for, 31-35

Position for cycling *(continued)*
  for climbing (uphill cycling), 66
  for interval workouts, 105
  for variable intensity workouts, 80
Preseason scheduling, 135
Progress
  methods for charting, 155-156, 157
  methods for checking, 29, 134, 139
Pulse rate. *See* Heart rate
Pumps, tire, 18
Purple zone workouts
  basic guidelines, 79-80
  specific instructions, 81-90
  summary table, 91

Q

Quadriceps stretching exercises, 44

R

Race-pace workouts (speedplay workouts),
  119, 124
Racing. *See* Competitive cycling
Rating of Perceived Exertion (RPE). *See*
  RPE (Rating of Perceived Exertion)
Reading stands, 18
Recovery. *See also* Rest schedules
  from orange zone workouts, 106
  specific zone workouts for, 53, 65
Red zone workouts
  basic guidelines, 119-120
  specific instructions, 121-126
  summary table, 127
Rest schedules, 52, 131-132, 136. *See also*
  Recovery
Rewards, 156
Road bicycles
  adjustment of, 33
  selection of, 12
Road race workout (speedplay workout),
  119-120, 124
Roads, choice of, 21
Roller skating, in-line, 150-151
RPE (Rating of Perceived Exertion)
  for blue zone workouts, 52, 65, 77
  for green zone workouts, 52, 53, 64
  methods for measuring, 51
  for orange zone workouts, 52, 105, 117
  for purple zone workouts, 52, 79, 91
  for red zone workouts, 52, 119, 127
  for workout zones, overview, 51, 52
  for yellow zone workouts, 52, 93, 104
Running
  compared to cycling, 8, 9
  guidelines for cross-training with, 147-148

S

Saddle bags, 18
Saddle height, 32-33
Saddle sores, 16
Safety. *See also* Fitness checks; Injuries
  cooling down for, 41-42
  eating for, 22, 66
  equipment for, 16-19, 22
  helmets for, 16
  hydration for, 22, 66
  laws for, 21-22
  location selection for, 21
  warming up for, 39-40, 105
Shifting. *See* Gearing technique
Shoes, 17
Shorts, 16
Skating, in-line, 150-151
Skiing, cross-country, 148-149
Smoking, in fitness assessment, 25
Speed, workouts for building. *See also*
  Interval workouts; Time trial workouts
  aerobic intervals, 93, 94-97, 99-102, 132
  orange zone, 110, 115
  purple zone, 87-89
  red zone, 124
  sample schedules, 140, 143, 146
  speedplay, 110, 124
  speedwork, 87-89
  sprints, 115, 133
  yellow zone, 94-97, 99-102
Speedplay workouts
  orange zone outdoor, 110
  red zone outdoor, 124
Speedwork workouts, purple zone
  outdoor, 87-89
Sporting Goods Manufacturing Association,
  4
Sprint workouts
  basic guidelines for, 106
  benefits of, 133
  orange zone outdoor, 115
Standing body position, 66
Stationary cycling
  benefits of, 4
  blue zone workouts, 71
  equipment for, 15, 18
  green zone workouts, 58, 63
  interval workouts, 105-106, 111, 116
  motivation for, 154
  orange zone workouts, 111, 116
  pedaling technique for, 79, 106
  purple zone workouts, 85, 90
  red zone workouts, 119, 126

simulating climbing (uphill cycling) with, 66, 79
steady ride workouts, 58, 63, 85, 90
time trial workouts, 103, 126
variable intensity workouts, 71, 76, 98
in winter training schedule, 135
yellow zone workouts, 98, 103
Steady climb workouts
  basic guidelines, 65-66
  blue zone outdoor, 72-75
  purple zone outdoor, 81
Steady ride workouts
  benefits of, 132
  green zone outdoor, 54-57, 58-62
  green zone stationary, 58, 63
  purple zone stationary, 85, 90
Stress tests, 50-51
Stretching exercises
  after cross-training, 148, 150
  basic guidelines, 40, 42
  benefits of, 41-42
  specific instructions for, 42-47
Swimming, compared to cycling, 8, 9

T

Target heart rate, determination of, 51. *See also* Heart rate
Technique, basic guidelines, 31-37. *See also* Gearing technique; Pedaling technique; Position for cycling
Tights, 18-19
Time trial workouts
  basic guidelines for, 106, 120
  benefits of, 134
  orange zone outdoor, 112-113
  purple zone outdoor, 86
  red zone outdoor, 125
  red zone stationary, 126
  yellow zone stationary, 103
Tire pumps, 18
Tools, selection of, 18
Touring bicycles, adjustment of, 33
Trails, choice of, 21
Training programs
  basic guidelines, 52, 129-130, 131-136, 137
  for beginning cycling, 130, 138-140
  for competitive/intense cycling, 130, 144-146
  elements of, 132-134
  for frequent/moderate cycling, 130, 141-143
  goal setting for, 154-155

intensity selection guidelines, 49, 51, 52, 130
log for charting progress of, 155-156, 157
modifying schedules for, 134
progress checks for, 29, 134, 139
rest in, 52, 131-132, 136
selection of workout zones for, 49, 51, 52
yearly scheduling for, 135-136
Triathlons, 4
Turning practice, 80

U

U.S. Cycling Federation, 120

V

Variable intensity climb workouts
  orange zone outdoor, 114
  purple zone outdoor, 82-84
  yellow zone outdoor, 96-97
Variable intensity workouts. *See also* Variable intensity climb workouts
  basic guidelines, 80
  blue zone outdoor, 67-70
  blue zone stationary, 71, 76
  yellow zone stationary, 98

W

Warming up
  basic guidelines, 39-40
  for interval workouts, 105
  for weight training, 150
Water bottles and cages, 18
Weight, body, and fitness, 25. *See also* Body composition
Weight training, 149-150
Wind trainers, 15
Workout zones
  blue zone, 65-77
  color-coding of, explained, 49
  green zone, 53-64
  intensity of, overview, 49, 50, 51, 52
  orange zone, 105-117
  purple zone, 79-91
  red zone, 119-127
  selection of, 49, 51, 52
  yellow zone, 93-104

Y

Yearly training program, 135-136
Yellow zone workouts
  basic guidelines, 93
  specific instructions, 94-103
  summary table, 104

About
the Authors

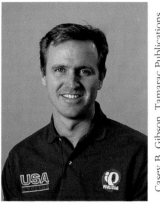
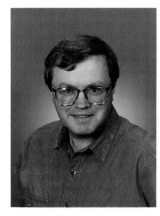

Casey B. Gibson, Tamarac Publications

Chris Carmichael   Ed Burke

With more than 20 years of cycling experience, including 5 years as a professional cyclist, Chris Carmichael has established his cycling expertise. He raced in the Tour de France with the first American team to participate and was a member of the 1984 U.S. Olympic Team. Chris has coached the National Cycling Team and the 1992 Olympic Cycling Team. He has served as the national coaching director for the U.S. Cycling Federation since 1993. His USCF duties also include overseeing the Athlete and Coaching Programs and the Olympic Preparation Department. Chris and his wife, Perrin, live in Colorado Springs, where Chris enjoys cycling, cross-country skiing, and cooking.

Ed Burke has written or edited seven books on the subject of cycling and is renowned for translating the latest scientific research into practical applications for cyclists. He coached the 1980 and 1984 U.S. Olympic Cycling Teams and was the director of sports science and technology for the National Cycling Team from 1981 to 1987. Ed holds a doctorate in exercise physiology from Ohio State University and is an associate professor in the Department of Biology at the University of Colorado. He lives in Colorado Springs with his wife, Kathleen.

Credits

"Assessing Your Cycling Fitness" on pp. 24-26 is from *Jog, Run, Race* (pp. 20-22) by J. Henderson, 1978, Mountain View, CA: Anderson World. Copyright 1978 by Joe Henderson. Adapted by permission.

Stretches and their descriptions on pp. 42-47 are from *Sport Stretch* (pp. 62, 70, 79, 90, 91, 96, 104, 116, 128, 131) by M.J. Alter, Champaign, IL: Leisure Press. Copyright 1990 by Michael J. Alter. Adapted by permission of Human Kinetics.

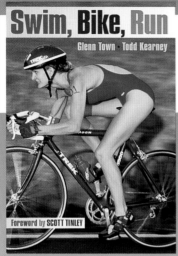
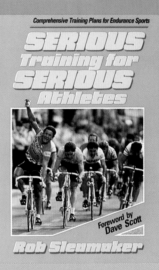